THRIVE BEYOND TRAUMA

Coach yourself to move on in a troubled world

Keith Nelson

Grosvenor House
Publishing Limited

Stanley, from Singapore

In the midst of global and individual upheaval, this is an important, timely work. Clear and compassionate, Keith's book offers a down-to-earth recovery methodology ideal for those from across the spectrum of trauma committed to healing. Drawing on decades of experiences coaching hundreds of clients, Keith makes use of an abundance of relatable, vivid – and often deeply personal – case studies to illuminate the range of possible paths for moving beyond the patterns of the past that all too often ensnare us.

Stanley Ng, *Founder & CEO, Sage Capital, Singapore*

Leonie, from England

Keith has walked beside me for many years as a phenomenal coach and mentor in my personal and professional life. Incredibly he has managed to transpose his nourishing and insightful presence into the written word through this wonderful book. Drawing on his vast experience of connection with others and bringing together years of research into understanding trauma, Keith has gifted us a beautifully intimate, accessible resource. Shining a light on the universal truth that everything we need to live an enriching and healthy life is within.

Leonie McCarthy, *MBE, England*

Aga, from Poland

I met Keith as Programme Director of the Cambridge Advanced Executive Coaching Programme at the Møller Institute at Churchill College, University of Cambridge.

The sessions with Keith and his approach to coaching raised my understanding of my role as coach, where the client, their transformation and the coaching process itself is the most important.

Keith is a calm and connected coach with great non-judgemental empathy. He has an incredible ability to reach the most sensitive areas. In a safe and attentive way, Keith can bring the client to the point – sometimes to a painful point – where the client changes their perspective and can often transform their life. Keith's full focus on the client's presence can take you where you didn't know you dared to go…

Thrive Beyond Trauma: Coach yourself to move on in a troubled world is not only a comprehensive study of trauma, but also a professional approach to coaching and a very useful coaching manual with tools, examples, and descriptions of real coaching situations. It is definitely a book to be studied and not just to be read.

Agnieszka Marek, *Executive Coach, Poland*

Gillian, from England

Keith is a gifted and experienced coach and writer, who brings his whole self to his work. During lockdown he used his time to diligently and selflessly research and write about his life experience around trauma so that others might benefit. Keith has deliberated to ensure this book shares truth and reality through a lens of compassion. He writes in an accessible and engaging style and includes real case stories which make the book compelling and provide a framework to support personal growth through trauma.

Gillian, *Executive Coach, England*

Francesc, from Spain

Meeting Keith Nelson at the University of Cambridge Institute of Continuing Education was the beginning of my inner transformation process through coaching. Since then, Keith has always been a key figure in my transformation process. It has been a journey where learning and change have helped me integrate a way of being and doing that aligns with coaching principles. Keith's holistic approach and calming presence have been essential in creating a safe environment in which I can develop professionally and personally. He combines kindness and professionalism, allowing me to explore all the aspects of my coaching journey safely.

Francesc Rubio, *Principal, Col·legi Mare de Déu del Carme, Spain*

Contents

Part 3: Acceptance 71

Trauma recovery stories: Karen

Part 4: Relief through release: why listening is so important 161

Trauma recovery stories: Rob

I believe it is important to tell and share personal trauma experiences no matter how difficult they may be. Untold traumas over time can make people feel small, invisible and almost non-existent. Healing traumas requires authenticity, courage and vulnerability. In this book, the reader will find eight different authentic stories or case studies which will help you see that you are not invisible and alone in your journey. After the stories come activities as well as hands-on advice drawn from different personal trauma experiences.

This is my first foreword. I decided to write it because, with the support of Keith as a teacher and coach, my life has changed. When I read this book, I realized that our personal traumas connected us. In addition, no matter how Keith and I are different as individuals, our reactions to events in our lives that we could not control were similar. Our traumas did not define who we are as human beings, but motivated us to find ways to work on ourselves and to make a difference in other people's lives.

As a survivor I think of the past events every day. I coexist with my trauma and I am proud of it. I am not a victim of the civil war, but a witness. I have a voice. I am heard.

As you read *Thrive Beyond Trauma: Coach yourself to move on in a traumatized world,* I want to encourage you to find the other voices in this book as well. Practice what it offers, and I believe that you will find yourself experiencing new possibilities, along with growing confidence that you can take on and succeed at goals that before were not imaginable.

If the trauma was a padlock, you hold the key to unlock it and thrive beyond.

Miroslav Miro Reljić

Author, speaker and resilience coach

Acknowledgements

I would like to thank Gillian for her empathy and support with the most difficult chapters in this book; Abigail and Toby for reminding me that no matter what happened in the past, there will always be a future; and all my clients for being my teachers.

This book could not have been completed without the many 'real life' stories printed here. They have been written by unique, beautiful people. The eight major case studies have been written by friends who are all wonderful people. It takes a huge amount of courage to share personal, traumatic experiences. Additionally, there are many smaller case studies, each anonymised and published with the agreement of the individuals concerned.

As these stories unfolded, I have appreciated, in wonder, not only how resilient people are, but how important it is that our individual, unique 'truths' be heard.

The truth does set you free.

Preface

Good can come out of trauma. It's often said that what doesn't kill you makes you stronger.

In researching, preparing and writing this book, I developed a number of beliefs about trauma, including the following:

- The long-term consequences of a traumatic event are frequently not fully understood or appreciated, either by the trauma sufferer or by their friends and families.
- Trauma is much more widespread than we might imagine. I believe that most, if not all of us, have experienced traumatic events in our lives.

Think, for a moment, about very challenging events in your life. Some of them might have happened and then faded away, experienced as difficult events. Others, however, might have left a traumatic impact upon you. This has certainly been the case for me, which prompted me to write this book.

In my work as a professional coach, I work with clients on an 'outside in' basis. It's through the strength of the coaching relationship that I support them to identify and achieve goals in their lives. They are on their 'inner' journeys. Reflecting on my own traumatic experiences allows me to write from an 'inside out' position. Sharing these stories – together with a series of case studies throughout this book – is a powerful way of learning how to recover from trauma. These stories remind us that we are not alone.

When working with clients, my aim is to create a relationship and a safe environment for them. Our work together often enables them to make transformational changes within their lives. Yet at the same time, I have noticed that some personal changes within me have been like mountains to climb. These mountains, confined to some areas of my life, would remain stubbornly unconquered for many years.

Looking back, I recognise there was a divide within me. On the one hand I was enjoying a successful and diverse professional career, yet on the other, there remained an unresolved and traumatised part of me. What I noticed in many clients, I also noticed in me. Technically the divide is described as dissociation, a word that is often used to describe a consequence of trauma. Very simply, in the middle of trauma, we might inadvertently cut a bit of ourself off from ourselves. Instead of being whole, we become divided. The trouble is, once trauma has passed, such dissociated separation can prevent us from joining ourselves back together.

The journey after trauma to health and wholeness can be a long and winding one. Public consciousness was raised with war veterans suffering from post-traumatic stress disorder (PTSD). Domestic abuse – mostly from men to women – has been another area to hit the headlines over the last few decades. And, of course, horrific abuse that is heaped upon children too. Trauma is also associated with events such as sexual assaults and murder, or huge man-made or natural disasters. We've all been living through one of these – the global pandemic.

Fortunately, most of us haven't been in the battlefields of military combat or experienced domestic abuse (although the statistics for abuse are shockingly high). But that doesn't mean we haven't been traumatised. I notice this when coaching clients. I meet people who show up for coaching as successful and healthy people who have good careers. Yet below the surface, many have been dealing with the aftermath of traumatic events. This is just a summary of the types of events and behaviours that colleagues, clients and friends have experienced in their lives:

- Sexual assault and rape.
- Daily beatings as a child in so-called 'care' homes.

- Shunned because of the colour of their skin.
- Lost siblings, either through illness or tragic accidents.
- Had parents who were absent, alcoholic, presented extreme behaviours and some who committed suicide.
- Family members who were murdered.
- Sexually predatory relatives.
- Whole families wiped out in terrible accidents.
- Married to abusive and/or coercively controlling partners.
- Experienced the onset of disabilities.
- Car accidents that have left their bodies pummelled.
- Accidents that left their ears permanently ringing with tinnitus.
- Had to make a terrible decision between staying with their violent husbands or leave and become outcasts from their own "community".
- Life-changing illnesses.
- Been sexually interfered with by people in positions of responsibility, such as coaches and teachers.
- Been brutally bullied by peers at school.

I could continue, but that is enough for now. Each and every example summarised above has emerged within conversations with individuals who are to all intents and purposes healthy, competent and capable people with good careers and families. Yet they have all experienced trauma up close and personal. And they were all going about their daily lives while doing their best to deal with their traumatic 'legacy'. Underneath the surface, they were working hard to keep things together. The consequences were there to be seen – whether it meant they moved to a different country, had spent time in jail, lost their jobs, decided not to have children of their own, or left their partners.

Trauma leaves behind a deep imprint. If you're one of those people getting on with their daily lives, while seeking to minimise trauma's legacy – the effects of which have a nasty habit of recurring – then this book is for you.

Additionally, there are the consequences of the pandemic, a traumatic event experienced globally:

- Losing a loved one – not being with them in their last moments; not being able to hug friends and family at their funerals.
- Coping with long covid.
- Losing job.;
- Losing businesses.
- Locked down during lockdown with an abuser.
- Struggling with social 'isolation'.

The purpose of this book is for you to untangle these challenges, to find your own path, to break free from the same old trauma tracks you might find yourself on. There is a huge amount that you can do. The case studies, advice and activities within this book are here to help you on your individual journey from isolation to connection; from dissociation to association; from disintegration to integrity and from separation to wholeness.

The journey beyond trauma is to move from surviving to thriving. To discard its unwanted legacy is a courageous and ultimately a liberating journey.

If you are reading this, then clearly trauma hasn't killed you. You are an ingenious survivor, and maybe you are stronger and more resilient than you think.

Keith Nelson

Prologue

Dressed in Personal Protective Equipment (PPE) from head to toe, the daughter sat beside her dying father. Curtains were drawn around them, cocooning them and separating them from the other bays in the ward. For her 83-year-old father, it was to be his last day on earth.

The ward, and others adjacent to it, were packed. All the patients, young and old, male and female, lay on beds, each and every one of them alive only because of ventilators by their sides.

Well, almost everyone. The father's ventilator had been removed, and he was moving towards his last breaths.

The Covid ward was remarkably quiet, as doctors and nurses went about their business professionally, diligently and empathetically.

The quietness and calmness belied a desperate scene, a place where the boundaries of life and death were so close. Just another day for the medics, who were months and months into this awful daily routine of dressing in their PPE, tending to the dying, risking their own lives, giving hope to the living and answering phone calls from anxious relatives unable to see their loved ones.

Father was a fighter. Twelve years earlier he had been given no more than ten years to live. Seven years previously he had been told he was terminally ill. He had fought on. The last three months had seen him deteriorate, and three weeks earlier he had been blue-lighted into the hospital.

It was there that he, and others, contracted Covid-19. What had been a non-Covid ward in the inner-city hospital became a Covid one.

Since Covid had been confirmed, it had been a tortuous time for the family, a rollercoaster of emotions. It was so difficult to know what was going on, and rare updates had given conflicting stories. It was cruel on the father, and cruel on the daughter and her family.

He was a resilient man and battled the illness. But eventually he succumbed, and it had been confirmed that the support would cease, and he would be allowed to pass peacefully and without pain.

The daughter had been told that she could be there for a maximum of 20 minutes. That was the protocol. Any longer and she would have to self-isolate for 10 days. But that paled into insignificance for her. Once the ventilator was turned off, life didn't usually last much longer than 20 minutes.

Seven hours later she was still with her father, being with him as she had been for the last few years, supporting him during his good times and bad times.

The doctor approached her and admired the father's resilience. "It happens," he said. "He is holding on for you. It's not unusual. He doesn't want to let go in front of you. When you leave, he will probably leave too." With that, the doctor wandered away.

The daughter paused, then turned to the compassionate nurse.

"Can I take my mask off and kiss him goodbye?" she asked.

"Yes," replied the nurse. "But only for a short while. Then you must go straight home, put your clothes in a very hot wash and scrub yourself from head to toe in the shower."

The daughter took her mask off and, kissing her father for the last time, she said her farewell.

Putting the mask on again, she walked through the ward. It was a traumatic journey past the ventilators, past the patients locked in their battles with the Covid-19 lottery before she was out of the ward.

Stripping off her PPE, sanitising her hands and face, she made her way through the hospital doors and into the darkness of the snow-covered car park, where she inhaled deep breaths of cold, fresh air.

Less than five minutes later her mobile phone rang. It was the doctor.

Introduction

The journey through and beyond personal trauma

The purpose of this book is simple.

To help you to cope with, recover from and ultimately move on from traumatic events and challenging experiences that you might have faced within your life.

I want everyone to live their lives in a very rich and fulfilling manner – and I want you to live a brighter future than might otherwise have been the case. After all, this is your birthright.

It's a journey that starts by becoming more aware of yourself. From this raised self-awareness, you are invited to explore new ways of being and create opportunities for action. It's a journey from how you live your life now through to how you might live your life in the future – and who you might become in the future.

Trauma comes in many forms. It's a fact of life that most of us have experienced traumatic or very challenging experiences. Once the traumatic event has happened, it's then up to us as individuals to cope as best we can.

The Covid-19 pandemic has been traumatic across the world. Dealing with its consequences will last for many years. The effects of this vicious, invisible, mutating virus have been felt at global, national, regional, local, family and personal levels. Countries fell out with each other, borders were closed, families were separated, and many thousands of people lost their lives.

One week, people were enjoying the freedoms of a liberal democracy. The next week, they were not allowed out, as lockdowns were sanctioned with immediacy and urgency.

We were told to stay at home and reduce or stop contact with others. Cafés, bars and restaurants were forced to close. Businesses ground to a halt. Schools and shops were shut. University lecture halls emptied. Airports fell quiet and planes were mothballed. Streets were deserted. People lost jobs. Countries took on enormous debts. Recessions hit. Millions died, as remaining family members sought to rebuild their lives under draconian conditions.

While this was going on, deep anxieties emerged – whether for health reasons, or finances, or isolation and future uncertainties – the list goes on.

Words such as self-isolation and social isolation were frequently heard. Think about those occasions when you have been distressed. A natural response is to seek out others for comfort, reassurance and often hugs and cuddles. But how could you seek out others for real and physical comfort when you were not allowed to meet?

We were forced to adapt to immense, life-changing regimes. A population that was suddenly told to live within the confines of its own homes. Reports of domestic, sexual and emotional abuse rose up far and away above the 'normal' levels. Thousands of women, children – and men – locked down within four walls with an abusive husband, parent or wife. The director of a mental health charity described the lockdown as "catastrophic". Awful, really, for many thousands of young people whose dreams and aspirations were halted in their tracks.

Disastrous for those with mental health problems or those who struggled to be alone. A real bruising for those people locked up with an abuser – whether physical or emotional.

Underlying this new 'normal', a real fear for this silent, invisible, lethal enemy. Something that could kill, but something that couldn't be seen, heard, smelt, touched or tasted.

It was a truly awful time, traumatic for many.

Trauma, as we shall discover, comes in many forms. The impact of Covid-19 affected so many people. Trauma is frequently experienced on a much more specific, individual level. There's a saying that every cloud has a silver lining, but to see those silver linings we need to be looking upwards, towards the sky. Too often the aftermath of a traumatic experience is a tendency not to look up, not to see opportunities.

As we shall discover, learning to look up is a journey, and that includes:

- Considering and accepting the impact of the traumatic and challenging events.
- Raising awareness of the effects of trauma.
- Creating a road map of activities that we can do, coupled with a sense of being, to loosen the grip that these challenging and traumatic experiences might otherwise continue to hold.

This book is designed to raise awareness and propose exit strategies for you to discover more of your potential and to move on and live your life more richly. The only person who can do that is you. The aim of this book is to help you on your journey.

Open yourself to a world of possibility

I am inviting you on a journey of personal transformation. This involves:

- Accepting yourself for who you are.
- Accepting what has happened to you.
- Focusing on how you can deal with it, what you can do and how you can be to create your better future.

It's important to understand what a traumatic event is and, crucially, to appreciate the full impact it can have upon you. It could be from isolation due to the pandemic; it could be the result of an abusive relationship; it could be the passing of a loved one, perhaps even a pet. By accepting, focusing and enabling yourself to move forward, you will:

- Become more aware of yourself, not only your mind but, crucially, your body.
- Tap into your inner resources and resilience.
- Explore your options.
- Make more effective choices in terms of being and doing.

I encourage you to keep yourself open to worlds of possibility, to enable you to bring more of your creative imagination to your life. Enjoy!

How to use this book

During the early stages of the first lockdown across much of Europe, I searched the words 'trauma' and 'news' on Google, and three headlines popped up:

- "Corona isolation prompts rise in domestic violence trauma cases…"
- "New mum recalls trauma of birth during lockdown…"
- "For some people, trauma symptoms won't surface until after the pandemic…"

Trauma is very widespread – and I believe that most people have experienced some kind of traumatic event during their lives. A traumatic event (or events) can be considered in two contexts:

1. The traumatic event itself.
2. The impact the traumatic event had.

Trauma can be experienced either directly or as a witness. Then there are the after-effects that people go on living with for days, months, years or even longer after the trauma was experienced.

This is where this book fits in. It provides you with greater awareness that the effects of traumatic experiences are having upon you. Then it explores ways of:

- Being and becoming more of yourself.
- Doing activities that will enable you to move forward.
- Loosening the grip that traumatic memories might currently hold over you.

Ultimately, it is designed to create an exit strategy for you from the traumatic after-effects and to show you ways to live a more satisfying and rewarding life. This richness can be experienced more fully within yourself, in relationships with others and within your environment.

I write this as someone who has experienced personal trauma. And as someone who has spent over 20 years coaching clients and listening to their stories. I've heard stories that have deeply troubled me. I have wept for my clients and experienced sleepless nights. I have allowed myself to be affected by my clients – which, for me, is part of the coaching journey. I process through supervision, meditative activities, calming music, exercise and other grounding activities.

And I have also marvelled at people's ingenuity, resilience, bouncebackability and fortitude in keeping going. My clients have been my teachers.

I have thought deeply about the impact that change has upon people. And I have reflected upon how people change and what prevents them from changing. Not only have I experienced their sense of being stuck in life, but I have experienced my 'stuckness' too.

Traumatic events often leave behind symptoms long after physical injuries have healed. Indeed, they can be carried for a lifetime. That evokes in me sadness and a sense of the unfinished. I like to live in a world of possibility and hope, of optimism and opportunity. Of the chances to move forwards – not just to a full recovery but to go beyond previous limitations to reach out for new opportunities.

It's crucial to acknowledge the traumatic or difficult event itself and the effect that the event has left behind on the person. It's hard to underestimate this. As will become clear, you don't have to be a war veteran or a victim of sexual abuse to suffer from post-traumatic stress disorder (PTSD). It is a combination of both the event and its legacy within the individual. And "disorder" is a strong word. Perhaps we can experience a range of effects that are on a continuum from mild to extreme.

This book draws upon both my personal and coaching experience. As a coach, working safely is crucial to my work. Consequently, I have invested in my personal development. To work safely and effectively, I regularly occupy the client's chair, sitting opposite supervisors, counsellors and therapists. With these people, I have shared my innermost experiences and thoughts. These also inform these pages.

I have also worked with body specialists too. From the subtlest of work with a cranial osteopath through to a physiotherapist who has sought to open my body up more widely and fully.

On my journey, I have come to realise that one of the greatest gifts we can give each other is so simple yet so important. Just listening. The simple act of being present for another and using listening to underpin the relationship.

Listening with our whole attention. Not talking, not interrupting, not telling, just listening as best we can and not judging. Accepting the person for who they are. Hearing and seeking to understand their stories. Allowing them the freedom and safety to offload, to cry, and then to notice what emerges on the other side of the tears.

Over 700 years ago, the Italian poet Dante penned *The Divine Comedy*. An allegory on human life, and placed in the Christian

Afterlife, the Roman poet Virgil guided Dante through hell and purgatory, while Beatrice, his lover, led him through heaven.

My spin on this is simple. Trauma can be hell on earth. It can be followed by many years – if not a lifetime – of purgatory, with flashbacks to hell.

And this is my invitation to you. I invite you to make your journey one of moving further and further away from hell and purgatory to a living 'space' in which you can claim – or reclaim – your right to live freely. My sense of heaven on earth as a concept (which is not a religious interpretation) is being at peace. At peace with oneself, at peace safely with others and at peace with the environment and the world.

I believe it is your birthright to live your life intimately, with autonomy and with spontaneity.

- Intimately: co-creating relationships with others that allow you to bring your full self to a relationship and to accept the other person that way.
- Autonomy: to live your life fully. To set your agenda, rather than have others (past, present and future) set your agenda for you.
- Spontaneity: to allow yourself to be free and live 'in the moment' and inhabit more of your natural, free and spontaneous self.

Growing up in life, it's too easy to lose sight of these. Traumatic and difficult experiences can have a huge impact on the ability to function intimately, autonomously and spontaneously.

So, let's go on a journey together to confirm our birthrights, help others to reclaim their birth rights and to live more fulfilling lives. Awareness, as we will discover, is crucial.

Let's explore this world of possibility together!

Disclaimer

There are many stories, chapters of advice and exercises that you can complete in this book.

The content of this book – which explores trauma and the impact it can have – might be challenging to read.

I encourage you to be your own thermostat here – if the chapters feel too much or the activities are challenging, then turn the thermostat down and walk away. Give yourself a break, step away. You might notice more about your triggers and the impact that the traumatic event might still be having for you today.

Step away, notice, let yourself breathe.

PART 1

Understanding trauma and its impact

Trauma is one of those words that has become very common in day-to-day language but is often simply not understood. It's relatively straightforward to accept that such events as wars, pandemics and abusive relationships can be traumatic. What is much more challenging to understand, however, is the impact that a traumatic event can have upon a person. Indeed, a significant frustration for someone who has suffered from a traumatic episode is that of not being understood by others.

We will start by seeking to understand what trauma is; then move on to a deeper understanding of traumatic experiences. The next chapter in this section describes a traumatic continuum from the mild through the substantial to the severe.

Finally, we conclude this section with a chapter on a particularly disturbing aspect of trauma – abuse. This chapter combines three elements.

- Firstly, a victim's story.
- Secondly, through the statistics, which are shockingly high.
- Thirdly, through the words of a former chief superintendent in the Metropolitan Police, who has significant experience of the shocking effects of abusive crimes.

CHAPTER 1

What is trauma?

A traumatic event is bad enough. Yet it's the impact it has on the individual that can be so devastating.

Typing the word "trauma" into a search engine returned 316 million results in 0.59 seconds. Trauma's a bit like that. Overwhelming and immediate. It can very quickly be in your face and, before you know it, absorbed into your body and mind too.

For some people, a traumatic experience can lead to PTSD. There is a charity, PTSD UK, which describes the defining characteristic of a traumatic event as:

"...its capacity to provoke fear, helplessness, or horror in response to the threat of injury or death".

Those words pretty well sum up the immediacy of trauma. A traumatic experience can lead to PTSD, and Aphrodite Matsakis notes that PTSD is a *normal* reaction to *abnormal* amounts of stress.

Follow this reasoning, and PTSD is less a mental health issue and more a response to intense adversity. Yet it can then become a mental health issue. When there is a traumatic or very challenging event, it's helpful to remember not just the event but also the individual's reaction (or response) to the event. How someone reacts suggests an 'automatic' reaction. Perhaps response gives a greater element of choice – and hence control.

Traumatic events come in many forms. These can be a single event or a series of events. It can be complex – with different factors involved.

Trauma has been described in a number of ways, including:

- Acute trauma, from a single incident.
- Chronic trauma, perhaps from a long, repeatedly abusive relationship.
- Complex trauma, from a variety of traumatic events. These are very personal and invasive.

It is helpful to break these down and consider events that might lead to traumatic reactions. The table below describes a number of these.

Serious accidents	This might be a car crash, for example. Or an accident at work. Or falling down the stairs.
Bereavement	Losing a loved one, which can affect all family members of whatever age. Sometimes very suddenly, with no chance to say 'goodbye'. Consider the impact of the death of loved ones during the pandemic, when there were very limited opportunities to say 'goodbye' (while they were still living), or appropriately mark their passing at a funeral.
Witnessing death	This could be a single death, perhaps of a family member or even a stranger. It could be multiple deaths – as might be the case for health or care workers – seeing multiple people pass away, particularly when the pandemic was at its height, and there were many deaths.
Military combat	Military personnel involved in or with others in wartime combat.
Terrorism	Being involved in or witnessing a terrorist attack. Notice both roles – as someone involved and as someone who witnesses an event. (Witnessing events applies to many of the trauma-creating events described here.)

Violent personal assault	Physical attack, sexual assault, burglary, robbery, mugging.
Disasters	This could be natural, such as an earthquake, tsunami or a storm. Or man-made, such as buildings collapsing, fires, or other such events.
Abuse	This can be prolonged over a period of time. Can be experienced in different ways – physically, sexually, emotionally. These can be either distinct or interwoven. Coercive control is a form of abuse. [It's important to remember that abuse doesn't need to be physical.] The majority of perpetrators are men, but not exclusively so.
Bullying	Exposure to bullying behaviour.
House fires	Experiencing a house fire.
Childhood neglect	Being neglected as a child.
Miscarriage	A miscarriage. (Impact on self, partner, siblings and siblings-to-be.)
A life-threatening illness	Being told you have a life-threatening illness.
Childbirth	Childbirth. Experienced either as mother, partner or siblings; perhaps even the baby itself. Or miscarriages, or still-born babies.
Operation	Reaction to an operation, large or small.
Refugees / asylum seekers	Journeys from country to country. Risking everything to be loaded into containers or boats to find a safer place to live.

This list can go on and on. Many of these can be found on the PTSD UK website. There is a very broad range of potential traumatic events. You may have experienced something that is not within the table above. It's not intended as either a prescriptive or comprehensive list.

Now comes the crucial point.

It's how the event is experienced and internalised into the body and mind that is really significant.

Let's imagine for a moment that you were bullied as a child. Even as an adult, it can stay with you. There is a danger that you might minimise – and attempt to mentally dismiss – the event. You might consider it insignificant alongside the experiences of a war veteran. But it is your world, your reality. And bullying is abusive. This might particularly apply if your traumatic experiences were when you were young – many years ago in the past. Such experiences can be locked away into the subconscious. Some of the mental challenges for you in this instance might be one – or more – of the following:

- Minimal or semi-awareness, lost in the subconscious. You're not fully aware of the extent of the impact that the event had upon you.
- You minimise it. It doesn't feel that significant. After all, lots of children were bullied.
- Just get on and do. You focus your attention on action – doing things to keep you occupied, physically and mentally.

Such minimisation – and ongoing bursts of anxiety too – might keep it manageable, but without it ever really going away.

It's also helpful to be aware of the impact of trauma as a witness. You might have witnessed another person's death. Or lain awake at night, quietly frightened or enraged while mother was being abused by father, or brother was being beaten by father, or sister was being raped by stepfather.

Yet if we attempt to keep the effects buried, minimise them, just try and get on, then the odds are severely stacked against them going away. It will be a burden throughout a lifetime.

But the good news is that the body and mind can heal. There is hope. As PTSD UK declares on its website: "Tomorrow can be a new day."

This is the time to create not just one but lots of new days.

The journey from the effect of a traumatic experience is about walking through new doors. It is up to you to open those doors. Only you can do it. This book is here to help. And remember this. You have the key in your pocket.

Chapter 2

Understanding trauma

You don't have to be a war veteran or a victim of abuse to experience traumatic events.

Say the word 'trauma' and many people's thoughts go to two things:

- Trauma experienced by soldiers in wartime.
- Trauma experienced by women in abusive relationships.

Because of our cultural norms, the *majority* in the first case tend to be men, while *most* of those in the second example are women. But, of course, not exclusively, which is often overlooked.

As we have seen from the previous chapter, a phrase that is commonly heard when discussing war veterans is PTSD. But this acronym is used much less frequently when talking about women who have been victims of domestic violence.

And PTSD is applied even less so in other situations and contexts. Remember that trauma can be experienced in lots of different ways, and its impact can remain for a lifetime. Its effects are internalised in both body and mind. Remember that our bodies contain our whole being, so expect psychological consequences to be absorbed into the body somewhere.

Its effect is often severe. It's the skilled therapists who *really* understand trauma – for the rest of us, it's easy to underestimate either its impact or its longevity. It's not unusual for others to expect the trauma 'sufferer' to move on. Indeed, they may become frustrated and sometimes even annoyed when this doesn't happen.

And they don't move on because they don't know how. It can be so difficult, with the effects of the trauma stuck away somewhere in the subconscious and within the body – perhaps it manifests through a tight chest or a knotted stomach.

Fans of *Jurassic Park* movies will remember those occasions when the characters in the film – often children – have those heart-stopping 'awareness' moments when they stumble across giant footprints left by enormous, terrifying dinosaurs. Over time, those footprints bake hard, leaving their indelible shapes stamped into the ground below.

Trauma is like that. The PTSD UK website estimates that one in two people will have a traumatic experience during their lives, and 20% [over 6 million people] can go on to develop PTSD. But even if you don't go on to develop full PTSD, you still have the memories inside you. This book acknowledges trauma experiences on a continuum: the memory of those experiences without necessarily having developed into significant PTSD. This is described in the next chapter.

Consider those baked-hard footprints. Imagine they trod on someone whose life after the trauma might then be experienced in various ways, including:

- Physically, with that footprint embedded somewhere within the body. It's as if something has been squashed, and sufferers may be (or may not yet be) aware of tensions and tightness within their bodies.
- Psychologically, for example through subsequent hyper-vigilance, jumping at a shadow in case it hides a lurking monster; and anxious, just not feeling safe.
- Emotionally tired, taking up a lot of energy just getting through life on a day-by-day basis.

That can all too easily become a reality. And a reality that seeps into so many aspects of life.

Armies used to fight battles in faraway lands, often taking weeks to travel from home to the battlefield. Nowadays, they can be transported from peace to war in a matter of hours. And brought back in just as quick time. One week, risking their lives facing an enemy. The next, dropping the kids off at school with the other mums and dads. And sometimes the battlefields far away have been less formidable than the challenges they face among communities when back home.

Few of us can be expected to comprehend what it is like to spend time living in a kill-or-be-killed situation. Or what it is like to be sexually abused, drunken night after drunken night.

For many of us, trauma is something 'out there' and a topic that most would rather not have to cope with. Consequently, it is left to the world of psychologists, psychiatrists and psychotherapists to diagnose and deal with. For trauma survivors, the traumatic memory can colour, accentuate or dull all their experiences. And then they struggle to work out what is happening and are perpetually walking through the mists and mysteries of unhelpful patterns of behaviour.

Imagine, for a moment, wearing a veil over your face. Every moment of every day. Everything you see is through the veil. It is a distorted reality. Your vision isn't clear; perhaps the sounds are ever-so-slightly muted. Your smell is dulled. Physical contact is reduced. If it covers your ears, then you hear a muffled sound. This can be an effect of trauma – a detachment from and struggle to be in the here-and-now. Awareness is distorted. It really can be a lifelong imprisonment. Consider this situation in reverse, too. If you can't see out clearly, what can others see of you?

The 19th-century poet Henry Longfellow wrote a poem about a girl who, "when she was good, she was very, very good" but "when she was bad, she was horrid".

It's a well-known poem, and I wonder how often those words have been repeated to young girls growing up around the world.

Hopefully those girls heard it safely and saw it just as a poem. But perhaps, for others, it has become part of their internalised belief system – that they are both very good and horrid. Perhaps that became their patterns. If you know the rest of the poem, the little girl was alone in the attic. Mother, mistakenly thinking it was the boys, rushes upstairs, "caught her unawares" and then "spanked her, most emphatic". So perhaps in later life that girl kept creating and recreating a series of hijacks in her personal life – to reinforce the consequences for having the audacity to express herself!

I do not intend to be overly dramatic with my hypothesis. Imagine that girl scolded repeatedly, with an abusive parent, who consequently learnt to shut down her emotions to protect herself. Imagine the possible challenges for her in future relationships if she is unable to access her emotions.

Perpetrators of abuse who have been convicted of crimes often have the opportunity for early release through parole. For their victims, however, theirs can be a lifelong punishment. Physical doors are easy to open. Psychological, emotional and physiological doors are more intractable.

And the pandemic might have introduced new 'variants' of PTSD. One of these has been described as PPSD – or post-pandemic stress disorder.

Research released in 2021 described the Covid-19 pandemic as a 'traumatic stressor'. The authors, Victoria Bridgland et al., noted:

> "Overall, we found that participants had PTSD-like symptoms for events that had not yet happened, challenging the nature of traumatic stress as a problem pertaining only to the past."

Of course, such research is in its early stages – much more will emerge in the years to come.

And this newer description of 'PPSD' might also combine with existing PTSD conditions. Trauma can be complex, chronic, only partially understood, or even misunderstood. Yet the human spirit is remarkably resilient and has massive potential to bounce back.

The pages in this book are designed to enable you to deepen your awareness and create your exit strategy from the effects of trauma towards a richer and freer life. To enable you to open your personal doors to:

- Become more aware of your body and mind.
- Lift your veils or whatever filters you apply to your experiences.
- Encourage you to consider where your personal doors are – and how to open them.
- Suggest routes to opening and going through those doors to greater personal freedom.

There's only one person who can walk through those doors. You.

And remember. The key is always in your pocket.

CHAPTER 3

Traumatic experiences: the short-term, the substantial and the severe

Good can come out of trauma. It's often said that what doesn't kill you makes you stronger.

My first draft of this chapter heading was this: Traumatic experiences – the good, the bad and the ugly. It made me reflect on the following question. Can good come out of trauma?

After thinking about it for a while, the answer was clear – yes it can. Many good things have come out of the lockdown. Pollution levels dropped dramatically, families were brought closer, people learnt to work from home and their managers in the companies they worked for (had to) trust them to do so. Families spent much more time cycling, walking and enjoying time together.

It gave many people the opportunity to re-evaluate their lives and bring about changes that were perhaps long overdue. And as we will explore later, there can be a great deal of post-traumatic growth (PTG) as well as PTSD. It is often said that what doesn't kill you makes you stronger.

But somehow the word 'good' didn't sit with me very comfortably. And neither did the word 'bad'. It felt judgemental. [As a coach, I seek to be non-judgemental.] The word 'ugly' just didn't seem right. It's a label; it pushes the 'ugly' to the edges, often something that many people avoid thinking about.

Instead, the short-term, the substantial and the severe seemed much more descriptive and gave credence to some scaling.

PTSD can be extremely severe. It's when individuals suffer from PTSD – whether it is diagnosed or not. A severe disorder to learn to live with and recover from. And PTSD is the area for psychotherapists and psychiatrists.

At the opposite end is the short-term. The effects are felt and sting, but then subside without leaving a longer-term legacy. Ultimately the event is experienced as difficult, but one that does not leave the person traumatised over the long-term. Allow me to provide an example. Not long ago, while sitting watching the activities in a seaside harbour, a car drove into me. The car was travelling very slowly, and no harm was done. Apart from feeling a little shaky for an hour, I was fine. That's a mild event, with a quick recovery.

Sitting in the middle is the substantial. Those challenges in life that have been experienced as traumatic and very challenging. Experiences with the opportunity of recovery but possibly without the need for therapy. As well as traumatic experiences, I would add those troubling and challenging events that affect all of us as we go through our lives.

While we might not develop PTSD, we can – and do – carry these within us for years or even decades as 'unfinished business', described later in this book. It's those memories of past experiences that stay – and interfere with – our ability to move forward as effectively and quickly as we would like. These cause us interference. These memories interfere with how we lead our lives – unless, of course, we become more aware of this unfinished business and do something about it.

This is an important area to consider. Let's scale it to see what it looks like.

Impact of traumatic and/or related challenging experiences		
Short-term	**Substantial**	**Severe**
Keenly experienced; recovery in a few days or weeks.	The memory of traumatic and other events has left a long and lasting impact upon the individual. They continue to affect thoughts and behaviours.	May lead to PTSD.
Type of intervention		
Self-recovery; perhaps talking it through with friends. Perhaps coaching.	Traditionally counselling and therapy. Increasingly emergent in psychologically-based coaching.	Therapy. Diagnostic work.

My personal experiences are this. Things have happened in my life that are located in all three areas. It's down to how I experienced them. There's a world of difference between coping with an event and succumbing to it. Sometimes, it hinges on our personal capacity to fight back or run away (flee) the scene. Problems started when neither of these – fight or flight – were enacted. As we shall see, these are far preferable to freezing or flopping.

The intent of this book is to help anyone along this scale. But, as I repeat elsewhere, to do so from a position to add value, to raise awareness. And definitely not to replace essential therapeutic work.

I strongly believe there is so much that we can be doing for ourselves on a regular, daily basis. And much of it is pretty straightforward to do, as we will explore later in this book.

Chapter 4

The awfulness that is abuse

When a child is upset or hurt, its usual response is to reach out to a parent for comfort – to be held. Yet the child that has been abused might retreat into a place of isolation.

I have dedicated this chapter exclusively to the subject of abuse. It's written in five short sections, listed below. Sometimes statistics don't reflect the human suffering. And sometimes human stories don't capture the sheer scale of the problem. I have combined them both. I have also quoted John Sutherland, who, for a time, assumed responsibility for the Metropolitan Police's Racial and Violent Crime Task Force. This unit picked up responsibility for the police response to domestic violence.

- Introduction
- Definitions: what is abuse?
- The survivor's story
- The statistics
- The policeman's story

Introduction

Abusive relationships are, quite simply, traumatic. We cannot underestimate the enormity of the problem of abuse that exists nationally and globally. It is truly awful. When you read the statistics, remember these are just the recorded crimes – there are many more incidents going on behind closed doors.

It is an appalling situation that, unless addressed, will continue through the generations. Let's start with reports published on the BBC website, citing the United Nations that described the global increase in domestic abuse as a "shadow pandemic", with so many people trapped at home with their abusers.

Defining domestic abuse.

The Crime Survey for England and Wales (CSEW) states that domestic abuse is not restricted to physical violence. It notes that domestic abuse can "include repeated patterns of abusive behaviour to maintain power and control in a relationship." CSEW cites the UK government definition of abuse:

> "Any incident or pattern of incidents of controlling, coercive, threatening behaviour, violence or abuse between those aged 16 or over who are, or have been, intimate partners or family members regardless of gender or sexuality. It can encompass, but is not limited to, the following types of abuse:
>
> - psychological
> - physical
> - sexual
> - financial
> - emotional"

The survivor's story

Marilyn Van Derbur, former Miss America, describes in her book *Miss America By Day*, how she was raped thousands of times by her father from the age of just five to 18. Growing up, she separated herself into a 'day child' and a 'night child'. She describes how, after kissing her boyfriend good night at the door, she would then go to her room, only to be violated by her father.

That's just one example. Now let's look at the numbers.

The statistics

For the year ending March 2020, CSEW showed that an estimated 2.3 million adults (1.6 million women and 757,000 men) aged 16 to

74 years experienced domestic abuse. It equates to 5.5% of the adult population – about one in every 20 adults. The police recorded a total of 758,941 domestic abuse-related crimes in the same year.

The first lockdown in England was legally enforced on 26 March, 2020. Lockdown was eased from mid-May. CSEW reports that the National Domestic Abuse Helpline recorded a 65% increase in calls between April and June 2020, compared with the first three months of the year. In the week after the easing of lockdown, Victim Support received a 12% increase in the number of domestic abuse cases they were handling.

CSEW states that: "increases in demand for domestic abuse victim services do not necessarily indicate an increase in the number of victims, but perhaps an increase in the severity of abuse being experienced, and a lack of available coping mechanisms such as the ability to leave the home to escape the abuse, or attend counselling".

A further statistic highlighted by CSEW was the 700% increase in the number of visits to the National Domestic Abuse helpline during April to June 2020, compared with the three previous months.

On a global level, a shocking statistic provided by the World Health Organization (WHO) concerns female genital mutilation (FMG). It estimates there are 200 million women alive today who have been cut. FMG usually takes place between infancy and the age of 15. It is ritualistic abuse on young girls. It is carried out for a number of reasons – described on the WHO website, which is completely opposed to its practice. Very simply, FMG is an example of abhorrent cultural 'norms' and 'traditions' that simply need to stop.

The police officer's story

John Sutherland was a chief superintendent in the Metropolitan Police. He's written an excellent book called *Crossing the line: lessons from a life on duty*. He cites statistics published by Her Majesty's Inspectorate of Constabulary (HMIC) which suggest that domestic violence and abuse account for more than one in 10 crimes committed. His view is that domestic violence should be prioritised over all other types of crime. He writes that "the harm caused by domestic violence has the potential to go on forever".

Abuse is endemic across societies and is truly awful.

Chapter 5

Keith's story: an unintentional trauma

Over the next two chapters, you can read my story. Events that happened in my life that were experienced either as trauma, or as just challenging or bad experiences.

In sharing my story, I hope to shed light on traumatic experiences and the traumatic journey. I have discovered that far too many people sit in silence, tied down by memories of the past.

The next chapter explores my trauma and the impact it has had upon me. The subsequent chapter describes why I decided to share my journey. I am a great believer in storytelling, and my hope is that my story may, in some way, help you.

An unintentional trauma

Understanding what makes an event 'traumatic'

Greece is famous for many things, but I don't recall being shot at as one of them. Yet it happened to me. I can still vividly remember the whoosh of a bullet as it flew past my ear. It had been one of those surreal experiences when time went in slow motion. I was out for a run, making my way across rough terrain in search of a beach. Approaching me was a man a hundred or so yards away from me, carrying a gun. He stopped, deliberately raised his rifle, pointed it at me and pulled the trigger. In shock, disbelief and fear, I turned and ran as fast as I could. I weaved to the left and right as I sped away, but luckily there were no more shots. It could have been a traumatic incident, but it wasn't.

Neither did it prove to be traumatic when I was mugged in Hartlepool railway station. I felt the blade of a knife pressed to the side of my stomach and decided that being robbed on a late Saturday afternoon was the lesser of two evils. I used my head, handed over what the mugger wanted, and survived intact.

Nor was it traumatic in a dark and deserted street near Millwall when three drunks attempted to carjack me. They aggressively forced me to stop and tried to get into my car before I drove off. As the lead assailant was on my car bonnet at the time, he fell off. I looked back through the rear-view mirror to see him lying in the road. I drove on a safe distance and called the police. They later told me that the lead assailant spent that night in the cells after trying to "re-arrange a policeman's face" as a police officer later described it to me.

I was a child of the 1970s and, growing up in school, everyone knew which teacher to avoid being alone with. He groped me too, but I wasn't cornered and escaped his clutches. He was eventually fired as a paedophile. Disgraced, he left the UK to ply his trade in the Far East.

Then there was the Volvo driver in south London who, having bought a packet of cigarettes from a newsagent, decided to head south down the northbound lane of the A23 dual carriageway. We collided head-on. My week-old Audi was a write-off, I ended up in hospital having x-rays on my neck, and he was convicted for dangerous driving. Again, it wasn't traumatic, although since then I have always been extremely vigilant (sometimes hyper-vigilant, I suspect) when cars have appeared suddenly at T-junctions to my left.

On another occasion, I dragged a fellow hiker, who was suffering from hypothermia, across the freezing, snow-covered January landscape of remote Iceland to the shelter of a hut. I saved his life, as did two other people who then body-wrapped him to keep him alive until he warmed up.

I remember my first job as an editorial assistant on a national magazine and being 'let go' by the managing director just two days after my boss, the editor (who had hired me), had been sacked. I remember his words to this day:

> "We'll give you a reference, but we'll have to say you're not up to the standard of writing for a national magazine."

Incidentally, I went on to edit the UK's largest and most successful all-sports magazine and enjoyed a long, successful and award-winning career in magazine publishing.

There was also the occasion when I was detained by the police entering Sri Lanka, dragged a drowning girl to safety from the deep end of Watford swimming pool, caused a punch-up between rival taxi drivers in Antigua; was robbed of my passport, wallet and worldly goods in Beijing; and even took to the back roads of Gambia to avoid police checkpoints.

Dramatic and challenging as these all were, none of them were traumatic experiences for me. Indeed, they were mostly life-affirming and character-building. At the time of most of these, I was either an adult or going through my teens. And, looking back, most of the time I had a choice – fight or flight.

My trauma was much closer to home. And it happened when I was four years old. That's when I froze.

My trauma

Let me start by sharing two stories from my early childhood – one involving a dentist, the other conducted under medical guidance at home.

I will write about the dentist first, because that wasn't traumatic – what happened at home was. They provide an interesting comparison.

Those of you of a certain age might remember the era when the dentists' primary task seemed to be to stuff as many mercury fillings as they could in / on / between / around teeth. I've only recently discovered the reason for this. Simple – the more gaps they found, the more fillings they did, the more money they got paid. Let's just say that my dentist had obviously worked out that he was onto a good thing. And he was a brute! My sister and I used to go every three months (yes, four times each year) for our oral intrusions. Let's just say that neither of us were short of mercury by the time he had finished with us!

And, it seemed, every child went through similar experience at that time. Certainly, us siblings were well used to it.

It was tough, it was very intrusive – but it wasn't traumatic. Sure, I now choose my dentists carefully, and I have continued to visit the dentist for six-monthly check-ups throughout my adult life. My parents were doing what responsible parents did at that time – they sent us regularly to the dentist. And we all shared the same dentist – so there was a great deal of 'group' involvement and acceptance of the situation. We were all in it together.

Now let me go to a different intrusion – and one that left behind different memories.

As a child, I remember that lovely moment of being pulled out of the bath in the evening, wrapped in a great big towel and being hugged by my mother.

Early evenings, however, were also medicine time. I was one of those children who had trouble going to the toilet. So, after being dried off, it was time for a spoonful of liquid paraffin, designed, I later learnt, to ease bowel movements by softening the stools. This went on for many nights. I hated the stuff. It's only in hindsight that I appreciate how frustrated my parents must have been.

Clearly it didn't work because more action was needed and my parents, with the best intentions in mind – and following the doctor's advice – decided it was time for an enema. I can only imagine that they were at their wits' end with my blockages.

Being just four years old, I only have two fragments of memory of being given the enema.

The first was suddenly finding myself in their bedroom and seeing a bucket of soapy water, rubber gloves and an ancient-looking contraption with an ominously large amount of black rubber tubing. A towel was laid out on their double bed.

Before I move on to describe the second fragment, I think I should explain that enemas were not uncommon at that time. I am sure quite a number of readers will have experienced this procedure as well. Indeed, when I searched the internet on the subject of 'enema', the search engine yielded nearly 9 million results.

The procedure is still very much in use today – often to deal with severe constipation and as a precursor to other essential actions. Severe constipation can lead to faecal impaction, and the NHS website (2020) writes that faecal impaction may be treated with:

- "stronger laxatives – prescribed by a GP
- a suppository – medicine you place in your bottom
- a mini enema – where fluid is passed through your bottom, into your bowel
- a healthcare professional removing some of the poo – this is not something you should do yourself."

My enema took place over half a century ago, yet it is interesting that even today the NHS guidance – as I interpret it – indicates that it is only the poo removal that should be done by a healthcare professional.

Of course, many enemas were – and are – routinely carried out at home. So technically there is nothing 'abnormal' in doing this at home, even today. My frustrated parents were just seeking to fix a problem, which was normal practice back then – and indeed to this day.

So, onto the second of my fragmented memories.

Face down, twisting my head to the left, screaming I was held down and the tubing inserted inside me.

Afterwards, nothing. Blankness. I have no memory after.

Many, many years later, I asked my sister – two years older than me – if she remembered anything. She told me she wondered what on earth was going on with the screams coming from upstairs. She ran up the stairs to the landing but was shooed away.

Job done. Well, not quite. I don't think it worked. But at least I was never given another enema.

So that was my unintended trauma. I'm not a veteran of war and I've not witnessed terrible things. And I certainly had a loving and caring childhood.

My trauma had no malice or negative intent. It was my concerned parents, under medical guidance, seeking to fix a problem to make me better. Yet it was, for me, an unfortunate event in my life. Consider the following:

- As we have already seen with traumatic events, it's not so much the event itself but the impact on the person being traumatised that takes its toll.
- An important factor is whether or not the individual can do anything about it in the moment. Fight or flight can provide

great escapes. I could do neither. It was just a single, swift event.

I was unable to fight or flee from either the oral and anal intrusions – but they left very contrasting legacies.

The intrusiveness of the enema sank into my subconscious for many years and became locked inside me, both body and mind. It created something of a divide within me. Yet it had positive effects too. I developed strong personal resilience and my own way of handling things.

For very many years, I was unaware quite how much of an impact it was having in my daily life – as a child, youth and as an adult.

I've since read that one of the ways of dealing with trauma is to remember back to who you were before the traumatic incident took place. That's pretty difficult when you are four years old because you have so few memories of life before then.

So that was the trauma. An action with well-meaning intent, yet with unintended consequences.

As I grew up, a couple of things always disturbed me, but I could never put my finger on them. As a teenager and then as a man, whenever I looked at photographs of me as a boy, I was overwhelmed by feelings of sadness. Every time I could feel the tears welling in the back of my eyes. It was as if I was looking at a lost boy. Yet I could never figure out why.

And why did I always feel different? It was as if my destiny was to walk a path less travelled. Friendships and relationships were difficult. It felt both a lonely and bumpy path. As I grew older, it also felt a noble and independent path at the same time. I wasn't one of the crowd. I knew that through life I would carve out my track.

Growing up, I remember I used to like completing jigsaws. I was methodical. I would start with the edges to create a frame and then work inwards. Probably as most people do. But my own life felt different. The pieces were fragmented and wouldn't fit together.

It was different to the experiences with the dentist, because of the part of my body it affected; because it was painfully intrusive, completely unexpected and because it was done only to me. It was isolating.

It was only much later in life, through therapy, that the pieces would make sense, that I would start to join them together. A journey that allowed me to draw together a holistic perspective of my past – and to create a new vision for my future.

The effects

I will start with the positive effects. As we explore elsewhere, as well as post-traumatic stress disorder (PTSD) there is also post-traumatic growth (PTG). So, what have been some of my characteristics as I progressed through life?

- There was a significant divide between my professional and personal life. Professionally, I developed a great career. This only affected a part of my life.
- I possessed massive amounts of resilience.
- I developed a huge amount of creativity. I created and edited market-leading national magazines, became a published author, photographed professional calendars and travelled the world.
- I was able to change my career, culminating in my decision to steer my working journey to becoming a coach and coach trainer.
- I have trained well over a thousand coaches in my career and take pleasure from sensing the ripple effects of the values and benefits of coaching. I genuinely believe that authentic, person-centred coaching changes the world for the better.
- As a coach, using my motto *there is always another way* to help others through seemingly impossible situations.

Indeed, this allowed me to realise my purpose in life – helping others to change their lives for the better.
- A tremendous empathy for others.
- I developed as a solid, competitive runner – oh, how I loved the freedom of running through the countryside. And running in competitions is remarkably democratic. First one over the line wins. No arguments.

Now I will explore the negative effects – the ones I have been working through. It's impossible to say how much of the following can be traced back to that event, but it seemed to harmonise with patterns that I can now recognise.

- By the time I was 18, I had massive amounts of self-loathing and chronically low self-esteem. (But so did – and still do – many young people.)
- I believed there was something wrong inside of me that needed to be got rid of.
- I was probably suffering from low-level depression.
- Personal relationships followed a tangled pattern.
- I felt responsible for others' (plural) happiness. If the family was unhappy, I believed it was my fault.
- I could only be OK if everyone else was OK.
- It was very difficult – perhaps impossible – to trust anybody.
- Physically, my left hip was always less flexible than my right one. I walked with an ever-so-slight limp. My back was also out of 'neutral' position and very slightly arched. I've never been able to mount/dismount a bike while it is moving; activities like the hurdles at school were impossible. For many years the muscles in and around my left buttock were tight and I would easily become cold in that area. My sense now is that during the intrusion I twisted to my left and backwards. And some muscles remained physically frozen.
- Ongoing stomach problems.
- I could recognise two sides to me. A successful businessman, writer and coach on one hand, and a little boy in pyjamas on the other.

I know that the incident when I was just four years old had an incalculable impact on my life. Firstly, incalculable in that its impact was massive. Secondly, incalculable in the sense that I can't figure out for sure how much of who I was to become was due to that particular event.

But what I did realise, particularly when in therapy and when I was seemingly punched every week with new insights, was this.

The revelations all made sense.

It was as if I was coming back to myself.

Becoming whole again rather than remaining the divided person; bringing back together the successful man in his business suit and the anxious little boy in his pyjamas. Fitting the pieces of the jigsaw together.

It also gave me a deep personal experience – and later understanding – of trauma.

Working as a coach became very rewarding. One of the most satisfying aspects of working as a coach is seeing clients make positive, transformational changes in their lives.

The paradox for me was my own 'blockages' – why in certain areas I wouldn't shift. It taught me the impact of trauma's grip. And, for many years, I was in that grip. For too long, part of me remained frozen.

There were elements within me that were un-integrated. It revealed to me how deep trauma goes. And how unaware I was of its impact. As I wrote earlier, it happened to me when I was four. So that was my life – and my sense of identity – as I have known it. I have discovered that integration is a wonderful life position to move towards and achieve.

The felt sense

As well as the psychological effects it had on me – which can be seen in the descriptions above, there were various physical effects too – some of which are also described above.

Predominantly these have been in my stomach. Allow me to explain. For many years I struggled with constipation – particularly if tense or anxious. Defecating is a one-way process. The sphincter muscles (and I understand that we have an inner and outer sphincter) are designed to push out. Giulia Enders explains that the two sphincters are related to two different nervous systems. She writes that the outer muscle is controlled consciously – we decide when it is appropriate (or not) to go to the toilet and the sphincter remains shut. She contrasts this with the inner sphincter which, she writes, "represents our unconscious inner world." If we repeatedly prevent our need to go to the toilet, then, she adds, "our internal sphincter begins to feel browbeaten."

The result, she writes, is constipation. I like the link that Giulia Enders makes between the conscious world and the unconscious inner world. It simply makes so much sense to me and is another jigsaw piece that helped to explain my years of stomach problems.

For me, that's an example of the felt sense – explored later in this book – of how tension is stored in the body. In order to release the mind, we need to release the body. To ease the grip over those overly tight muscles. For decades I experienced, in certain situations, a very deep ache in the lower part of my abdomen. Not all the time, but something I grew very familiar with. My more recent focus has been to notice it, to become more aware of it – and the more that I have done that, the more it has faded away. To experience it now is the exception rather than the rule. It is much better now. A bit like the rest of me, it's work in progress. [As I believe we all are!]

Being understood

As I write later in this book, being empathised with and being understood is so important in the journey. For me, therapy was a crucial moment. Just to be heard, safely, just to be understood. To be validated. For years I wasn't, and I was in no position to validate myself.

Below are three conversational snippets that typified how difficult it can be for well-intentioned friends – and a social commentator – to describe it in their terms without 'getting' what it was like.

Firstly, the friend who said about parents and enemas:

"That was what they did back then."

That's very true, but at the time, her words just bounced off me. Then there was the second person who said:

"I had a friend who was given an enema, and she's alright."

In this example, I just sensed a lack of comprehension. I wanted to tell the person to politely go away. Yet there is good learning in this. It's how the traumatic event is interpreted that is crucial to understand. Imagine, for a moment, a mother and her five-year-old daughter. The mother is tired and feeling harassed. The daughter is demanding her attention every few minutes. In a moment of anger, the mother says, "Go away." How is that interpreted? On the one hand, just to:

- "Go away" (to the playroom) and play by myself or
- "Go away" (mummy doesn't love me).

The third was a conversation on *Yahoo Answers*. A teenager wrote about being given an enema and described his feelings of utter awfulness and devastation. His words absolutely resonated with me. Then came the comments. Some were supportive, but one commentator wrote:

"Suck it up, buttercup."

Not the most helpful sentiment ever written, but not unusual.

What happened to me was a dissonance between intent (make me better) and impact. I don't know if it was necessary. Who knows? If I hadn't had it, then perhaps I might have ended up in a worse state, maybe in hospital.

The experience has also humbled me.

I sometimes think about what it is like for children – and adults – to be intentionally sexually abused by their parents or partners. To be someone else's plaything. To have to endure those repeated intrusions that leave them as a ragdoll. It's then that I almost despair for our lack of humanity to each other.

And, of course, those abusers are often just repeating the cycle of abuse; on many occasions simply recycling the violence to which they were subjected.

Let's also not overlook the impact of the accidental trauma, which I experienced. Peter Levine describes how gynaecological procedures, abortions, enemas, thermometers and various "invasive surgeries" can potentially have traumatic consequences.

Coaching others has allowed me to move closer towards my life's purpose. To help others make real, positive changes in their lives. To live more freely and to achieve their goals. To support them to change their lives for the better.

And I learnt a crucial lesson in my training as a coach.

That I couldn't rescue other people, only care for them. Because if I was seeking to rescue them, I was really only doing it to rescue myself.

I don't know what challenging or traumatic events you have experienced in your life. Whether as a child, or as a result of the pandemic and lockdown. If this book helps you, inspires you, energises you on your journey, then it has done its job.

I hope my story helps you. I work as a coach. I write from my perspective of someone who has coached others *and* someone who has spent many long hours working on my own 'stuff'.

The focus of this book is dedicated to helping you to live your life in richer and more fulfilling ways. Ultimately, that's down to you. And if, as you are reading this, you are thinking 'suck it up, buttercup', then I suggest you consider taking this book to a charity shop and go and do something else that will give you more satisfaction.

Above all, there is a key thread that runs through the recovery from traumatic and challenging events, and I can describe it in one word.

Awareness.

It is only through self-awareness that we can really change.

- Awareness is curative.
- Awareness of yourself, others and your environment.
- Awareness of what has happened.
- Awareness of how you react – and then respond – to others.
- Awareness of how you show up to live your life fully each day.
- Awareness that your journey might take you to open new doors as you create your better future.

Remember, the key for those doors is always in your pocket.

Chapter 6

Overcoming my anxiety to write about my trauma

Why I needed to get out of my own way to write my story

Writing my trauma-related story in the last chapter evoked anxiety in me. Should I include it in this book? Or would it be best left out of this self-help book, which is really for you, the reader. This anxiety boiled down to a simple dilemma. On the one hand, not wanting to dishonour or disrespect my loving and caring parents, who wanted the best for me. On the other, wanting to share my story to help others. My intent in including this story is to write my truth – and for you, the reader, to understand and appreciate the fact that it was an unintentional trauma. As I mulled over this dilemma, I realised that explicitly stating this position was the only way I could complete this book.

After a long time of chewing my story over, I chose to share it. I decided not only would I write about my traumatic journey, but I would also share my thoughts and feelings around writing about this – in short, my anxieties. It's one thing to discuss topics with a therapist in a meeting room. It's another to publish it in a book. Keeping our anxieties to ourselves and hidden keeps us contained in a type of 'safety'. Sharing our stories involves risk. It feels less safe. Paradoxically, by sharing those stories, we create a new, larger personal comfort zone. It is only through coming to terms with my anxieties that I have become able to share my story.

To return to the purpose of this book, my aim is to help you to move through your life more effectively. And I am very aware that stories and storytelling are very helpful on this journey, which is why I chose to include my story, together with those of others.

I am confident in assuming that if your life has included difficult experiences – whether traumatic or not – then it can sometimes feel very difficult to get those experiences out in the open. It can be a challenge for us to be comfortable enough to feel sufficiently safe to disclose our innermost thoughts, our vulnerabilities, to others.

My intent is that by sharing my anxieties in this process, it will help you on your individual journeys too. Anxieties can take us over. Anxiety can be influenced both by deep concerns about the future and by our past histories, with the potential to freeze us in the present moment.

Hence paralysis, immobility, and just ending up feeling stuck.

In the previous chapter, I described how I was mugged in Hartlepool railway station. Many years later, when I returned to Hartlepool, I drove and went nowhere near the station. Was that a coincidence or my subconscious at work?

Consequently, I now realise, the bigger journey becomes that of overcoming anxieties. Allow me to explore my anxieties – and what I have done to overcome them.

It wasn't a big issue. In the scheme of things, having an enforced enema didn't seem a big deal. I might have been that one kid out of 10 who it affected. The other nine might have been fine. As the friend said to me, it is what people did back then. It doesn't directly compare with combat in war or repeated sexual abuse. **How I overcame this**. It was an intrusive event, and I was only four at the time. And I realise now it's *how* we experience events that matters. And my age when it happened made it a big issue.

I didn't want to be seen as a victim. In psychology terms, I couldn't countenance being a victim. It was, in my mind, 'weak'. I coach people about personal responsibility and not being caught in the drama triangle of persecutor, rescuer and victim. **How I overcame this**. Accepting myself as a victim proved to be a great relief and a release. A turning point into recovery and healing. By acknowledging myself as a physical victim, I became much less of a psychological victim. Only then could I stop being a victim. It was a liberating moment to appreciate this.

I didn't want to be judged. Writing and publishing a book is a very public experience. I found myself not wanting to be exposed to judgement. In my mind, those judges could be those anonymous, vicious commentators on social media; internalised figures in my head; and those people who just wouldn't get what my 'fuss' was about. **How I overcame this**. Age and maturity. I realise in life that I will connect with some people and not others. And vice-versa. I'm not on this earth to judge you, and you're not on this earth to judge me. If you do judge me, then it's your issue, not mine.

It felt disrespectful to my parents. The impact of what happened were the unintended consequences of a mother and father who didn't want to see their small son in pain and discomfort. But they put their trust in medical 'experts' – the mercury-mad dentist and the doctor who recommended the procedure. I had many happy and loving times growing up in a safe, caring family environment. **How I overcame this**. Both my parents have passed, and I explored this in therapy. I reflected on their childhoods and what had happened to them in their lives.

Dad flew in Lancaster bombers in World War Two. Out of 125,000 air crew in Bomber Command, over 57,000 (a 46% death rate) were killed in action. He saw colleagues from the squadron fly out, never to return. He saw the flickering flames of burning cities from the air. In 1945, shortly before the war ended, he was preparing to fly to Asia to continue the war against the Japanese. It never happened. Hiroshima and Nagasaki fixed that 'problem'. That was my dad's stark reality as a young man.

Mum was evacuated during the war. She was dispatched from London to Northamptonshire, aged eight. It is said that children who remained in London during the Blitz fared better psychologically than those who were evacuated. Imagine what it was like for a moment. Separated from your parents, living with other people, all the lights off during the frequent blackouts. In those days, they didn't have counsellors and therapists to talk things through with. They came from an era of just getting on. And as my friend said, it was what they did back in the day. Understanding their context is so important.

My parents simply wanted the best for me.

My shame and disgust. I felt a lot of shame. It was as if there was something wrong with me that needed to be got rid of. This was my shame, my secret. **How I overcame this**. Telling the therapist about this felt like a confession. And his words to me: it's how sexual abusers work; it becomes a secret. (Incidentally, it had become my secret without anyone telling me to keep it secret.) Writing in this way – and sharing this – helps me and, I sincerely hope, helps you. Let's get more things in the open. Truth sets us free, even if it does feel risky.

Feeling responsible. I grew up feeling responsible for the family's happiness or unhappiness. It was my fault when things went wrong. **How I overcame this**. Reframing my responsibility. It wasn't my fault. My sense of responsibility now is to help others on their journeys. Their journeys are their journeys. Learn from my experience and let's make the world a better place.

Feeling isolated. Loneliness and isolation can result from such events. For me, it was easy to withdraw myself – and observe. (Perhaps that's a reason that I became a writer.) **How I overcame this**. Discovering the power, value and benefits of relations with others, either professionally with a therapist or personally with loved ones.

Fractured sense of self. That split self of the professional businessman and the boy in his pyjamas. Holding those tensions and wanting to do the right thing. **How I overcame this**. Uniting the two aspects of self into a whole. From dissociation to connection. That makes me stronger. I am me. I am whole, I am integrated. I am OK.

Dealing with overwhelm. Struggling at the bottom of the deep, dark well. **How I overcame this**. Humour: being able to get into the here and now of lightness and not taking everything as the be-all-and-end-all. Very simply, planting my feet on the ground and learning to breathe into and out of my body. Noticing my body – attending to the pain deep in my lower abdomen to let it dissolve.

Letting go and forgiving. Letting go of the past and forgiving had the effect of loosening the knots that have bound me to the past. Forgiving others and forgiving myself. **How I overcame this**. As I write above, crucial in this journey was understanding context. Many people blame their parents for their woes. Yet understanding one's parents' context helps to explain many things. As I wrote earlier, they had their challenging wartime experiences, whether watching the bullets from the enemy's positions flying upwards in the night-time sky or hunkering down in the dark as enemy bombers flew overhead. And they put their faith in the medical experts. As a short aside, my grandfather on my mother's side fought in the First World War. He lost two brothers. He was luckier; he was shot in the testicle – and that tells me how fortunate I was to have been born in the first place. Looking back, understanding my parents' (and their parents') histories is so important in understanding their context for me – and consequently my context.

Being grateful. Learning to be grateful, not angry, was key. **How I overcame this**: I am grateful for a good upbringing and two kind and loving parents. I am grateful for what they did. Many benefits emerged as my life developed. It took me into coaching, and I developed a deep compassion for others. It gave me a gift of empathy. And as a coach, it is empathy for others that stops us being voyeurs into our clients' lives. At the end of the day, it enabled me to discover and actively follow my life's purpose.

Working out how to break a pattern. One of my values is speaking with integrity – telling my story so that I am heard and others can learn. Another of my values is around my family – as written above, not wanting to disrespect my parents. And there are also my daughter and son – now both adults. I have that impulse to want their lives to go beyond my own. Writing about this was a challenge.

Yet by sharing this story, I hope that they have a greater understanding of my context. After many years of not feeling I had a choice, I am now exercising my choice – to speak out. In doing this, my aim is to give them more choice and to break unhelpful patterns from the past.

I also hope that my story might benefit those in the medical profession who might be overly-focused on the physical issues, and less appreciative of the psychological consequences.

A turning point for me was being shown an excerpt from Ken Graber's book *Ghosts in the bedroom: a guide for partners of incest survivors*. He writes:

> "Other physical acts that become sexual molestation are… intrusive or unnecessary enemas and excessive personal involvement in toilet training."

That made so much sense to me. I remember sitting up all night to read his book. That was the starting point of validation of my experiences and feelings – very simply, my shame. What happened to me wasn't deliberate, but it had many consequences. Just as it was an enema for me, it could have been one of a countless number of medical procedures or investigations that are carried out on a daily basis on both girls and boys, and on women and men.

There you have it. That was my journey towards writing about my trauma.

I sincerely hope my words help you.

And I discovered one thing which I keep advising you to remember throughout this book.

I had the key in my pocket all the time. I just needed to know it was there, then find it, unlock the door, walk down the corridor and into a freer, more fulfilling life.

I invited you to learn from my experiences and remember: you always have the key in your pocket.

Thanks for reading my story about how I became 'OK'.

Part 2

Ignite the spark to get moving

Just as a fire needs a spark to get started, so we all need our own individual sparks to access our own resources.

Those resources are there, just waiting to be ignited. Over the next two chapters, we will explore ways in which you can consider how to create a spark that works for you.

Take a moment to think about so many things in life that are often taken for granted. To cook a meal, you need to buy the ingredients. To drive a car, you need to put fuel in the tank or charge the battery. To have a bath, you need to fill it with water. To go away on holiday, you need to travel to your destination.

Much the same applies here, except we also have a lot of choice.

To go out to dinner, you have a choice to get dressed for the occasion. To go to yoga, you can choose to buy yoga kit and your personal mat.

If you have ever had a flat battery in your car, then you know one solution is to fix a set of jump leads to your battery and charge it from another car. And the good news is that we're cleverer than cars. We have the capacity to start our battery from within.

Let's see how we can start to do this.

Chapter 7

Access your inner resources

We can pay a high price for trauma.

There are reasons why you picked up this book or chose to download it. Curiosity about the topic, the cover picture, a desire to deal with your unfinished business and to resolve trauma – perhaps a host of reasons have combined to inform your choice. It indicates that you want to make changes in your life. And, indeed, you are ready to do so.

Purchasing this book is a step. It shows how you are already accessing your inner resources and making decisions to move forwards. Progress is built upon many steps, whether large or small. And often that's how we all make a start – with small steps. The mightiest rivers start off as the smallest of streams.

Overcoming the effects of traumatic experiences can be a significant undertaking – often starting with (seemingly) small steps. Unhooking yourself from the tethers of trauma takes some time – because its impact can be so dramatic.

Trauma can be complex – as can the unpicking of its effects. If you celebrate Christmas, have you experienced that moment in the run-up to the big day when you unpack the Christmas lights and they are seemingly impossibly tangled? Patience, care and time are required to straighten them out. But sometimes you don't know where to start with that tangle of wires, which has been up in the attic all year. Traumatic memories can be like that. And then if you manage to untangle the metres and metres of wires, you plug them in – perhaps they don't work, or perhaps some of the lights are not working.

Judith Herman describes a range of trauma syndromes, such as hysteria, combat trauma, complicated post-traumatic stress disorder, multiple personality disorder and traumatic disorders. My sense is that its effects can influence every cell in the body.

There are excellent therapists who can help you through this work. I am not claiming to provide or replace therapeutic work. That is the realm of the specialists. I am a professional coach, and I work within the psychological, emotional and physiological arenas with my clients.

What I have come to appreciate is that, as we go through life, most of us will experience traumatic episodes to a greater or lesser degree – it is inevitable.

Accessing specialist therapy treatment is not always easy – or inexpensive. An individual might have access to a set number of Cognitive Behavioural Therapy (CBT) sessions through the NHS. Or through private insurance. Or people might just choose to pay for therapy. Such therapy is often a luxury for many – spending perhaps anything from £50 to £250+ for weekly one-hour sessions. Over the course of 12 or 18 months – or even longer – that adds up to a lot of money. And that can be off-putting.

But then again, what price can you put on your mental health as you progress through your life?

Look and notice within

The good news is that there are many resources available to us all – and mostly these reside within us, and often through our support networks.

We are, after all, wonderfully resourceful and resilient as individuals – and so many answers lie within. While few of us will spend any time in our lives in combat zones, for example, we will experience events that happen to us that are, to greater or lesser degrees, traumatic. A car accident, the sudden death of a loved one, or being put into lockdown with an emotionally abusive partner – the list goes on. And remember two things:

- Significant events will happen in your life that will be experienced as difficult or even traumatic.
- Even though your healing resources may not be immediately visible, they are there. The key is to make them both consciously 'visible' (through awareness) and viable (through making choices).

The awareness-based themes and activities described here can be applied to help you to move forward with your lives, to support you to:

- Access your inner resilience.
- Enhance your inner resources.

I invite you to tap into your inner world, your inner strengths, your inner creativity, your inner wisdom. My purpose is to encourage you to increase your awareness through:

- Increasing awareness of the impact of change.
- Increasing awareness of your body-mind.
- Increasing your ability to notice yourself.

And from these, to offer more choices and opportunities going forwards:

- Consider how *you can be* in your life.
- Suggest options for what *you can do* moving forwards.

Imagine on life's journey that you are driving a car and you have an accident. The following scenarios unfold:

- It is a minor accident, and both you and the other driver are pleasant and exchange details to resolve the issue via insurance companies.

- It is a more significant accident, and your body has had some bumps and bruises, but the other driver is pleasant.
- It is a minor accident, and the other driver blames you and becomes aggressive.
- It is a significant accident, your body has some bumps and bruises, and the other driver blames you and acts aggressively towards you.

These are all stressors and have the potential to impact you to a lesser or greater degree. Think through how you might react in all these scenarios. Add to it other reactions. Perhaps you're one of those people whose default mode means they automatically feel responsible – or maybe not. Or you are worried about telling your partner, or you blame the other driver.

Different people will react differently, with varying degrees of anxiety (from little or none to extreme).

The words here are written to help you raise your awareness so that you are more capable; firstly, to resolve old issues that lie within you and, secondly, to handle potentially challenging events in your future.

There is a saying that:

If you always do what you've always done, then you will always get what you've always got.

Let's add to that:

If you always react how you've always reacted, then you will always end up feeling much the same way.

Is that really a pattern you want for the rest of your life? I encourage you to:

- Be more aware.
- Do differently.

- Become more.
- And respond rather than react.

The choice is yours!

Chapter 8

When is this going to end? What you can start to do. Right now

Think about the control and influence you have over your life. It may be more than you imagine.

There are many concerns about the long-term effects of the pandemic. The psychological, emotional and bodily effects will be felt for many years to come. And that applies to future generations too.

To describe a few, these have included: having to socially isolate (I prefer the term 'physically isolate'); feeling trapped; feeling helpless; lack of human contact (on Zoom, WhatsApp, FaceTime and other video platforms we can see and hear, but not touch or hug); loneliness; fear of catching the virus; fear of (vulnerable) family members getting sick; the inability to live a 'normal' life; grieving and loss for major lifestyle changes; job losses; financial uncertainty; rising debt; anxiety over the national and global economic impact; kids not being able to go to school; not being able to do those things we took for granted; loss of loved ones; concern about going outside and leaving the house; being locked down with an abuser; depression; anxiety over not knowing when all this is going to end. It's a long list.

So much uncertainty, leading to anxiety and stress. Some people who hadn't previously experienced trauma were deeply affected by the crisis. By contrast, there were others who had previously experienced trauma who coped well.

As we shall explore, we can experience different reactions to traumatic events. Think of the fight / flight / freeze (or flop) responses.

Some people have fought the lockdown – they went on mask-free protest marches. Others wanted to flee the lockdown and travel to their havens. (But often not able to do so.) Others have accepted it – and perhaps become very accustomed to the rigid rules and regulations. Some might have frozen – struggled to know what to do – while others flopped and then found it difficult to start to move forward by going out again.

It was – and is – down to each individual to find their own way to cope with the situation. And it is important to remember that we can only control what we can control. There was a time when I could not control the fact that supermarkets insisted on people standing two metres apart, and I could not control the length of the queues to get in. But I could control when I chose to shop (to lessen the waiting time); I could choose a different supermarket to shop in; I could control whether to sanitise my hands and the purchases afterwards.

Taking more control can be achieved in many ways – as we will explore in this book. These are some of the more immediate things you can do:

You can:

- Set long-term goals to lower your uncertainty.
- Identify and create new habits.
- Generate routines that work around you.
- Create support systems.
- Trust yourself that you can adjust to new ways of living.
- Keep in good contact with trusted and valued friends and family members.
- Explore and connect online.
- Create new acquaintances and friends.
- Take up new hobbies.
- Find new activities to grow personally.
- See a therapist online or in person.

Here is an activity that you can try right now to become more aware of those things that you can control and those things that you can't.

Activity: extend your control over your life

You can make notes in this book, or you might find it easier to use a sheet of A4 paper for this. Draw three circles on the paper, as shown in the illustration.

- In the centre circle, write down things that you have complete control over.
- In the middle circle, write down the things you have some control over.
- In the outer circle, write down those things that you have no control over.

The purpose of this activity is:

1. To become aware of those aspects of your life which are within your control and those that are not.
2. To consider how you can expand those aspects of your life that you have some control over and to expand those things you have complete control over. And thereby diminish those aspects of your life you have no control over.

You might start by looking at your whole life or generate different circles for different areas of living. The example introduced above, about supermarket shopping, provides a useful illustration:

No control: Supermarket opening hours; supermarket guidelines/ rules; numbers of people allowed into the supermarket at any one time.

Some control: Staying two metres apart from others (also depends to some degree on others); when you choose to shop.

Complete control: whether you choose to shop in the supermarket or perhaps have online delivery; which supermarket to use. Using mask or visor, gloves, sanitiser. Cleaning the purchased products.

Increasing the size of the inner circles and reducing the size of the outer circle achieves two important things.

- Firstly, you become more aware of those things that you can influence and have greater control over.
- Secondly, you then give yourself the choice over whether or not to exert that influence or control.

The choice is yours.

Throughout this book there are different activities for you to try, each of which is designed to enhance you and your life as we all adjust to and then cope – and thrive – in the new ways of living. And there are many suggestions for how you can just 'be'. It has been called 'being in becoming'. Allowing you to be more of yourself in order that you can become more in the future. Ultimately, this can become a transformational journey.

Finally, I suggest you read the quote at the start of this chapter again. It's less about having complete control over everything. (None of us have this – and would we really want it?) It is more about the journey to integrating a more assured and stronger sense of self, to better cope with and respond to the ambiguities and uncertainties that life brings.

The dotted lines encourage you to consider how you can expand your locus of control

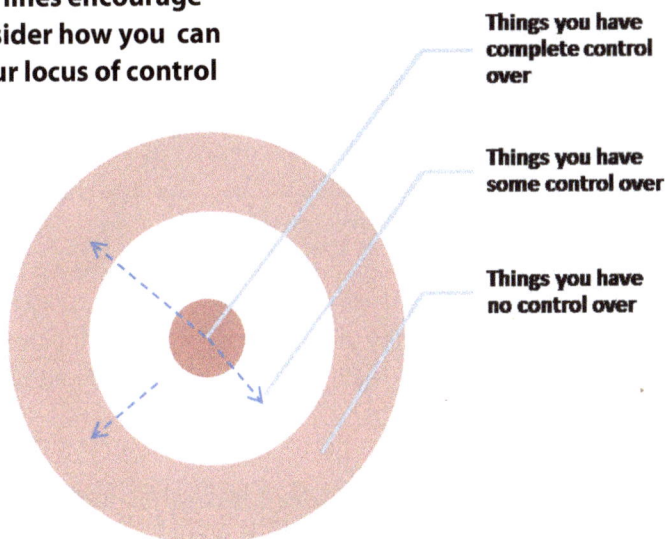

Things you have complete control over

Things you have some control over

Things you have no control over

Chapter 9

Time to get moving!

Traumatic memories in your body and mind are like old photos stored on your smartphone. They may be tucked away with thousands of other pictures, but they are still there.

One of the biggest problems with having the effects of trauma trapped within the body is that you can just carry on repeating old patterns and experiencing familiar anxieties. Curiously we have the capacity to create new pictures, but all too often the old ones keep recurring. We want to enjoy new images, but the old photos won't go. It's as if we sense we have the capacity to release ourselves from trauma's grip, but don't yet have the capability to do so.

Talking helps enormously but talking alone might not cut it. Indeed, speaking about the trauma might recreate it in a repetitive cycle. Discussions with friends can feel like that. Repeatedly going over the same things, feeling like the washing machine that is going round and round, seemingly endlessly.

There might not be sufficient awareness or energy to grab hold of the key that is always in your pocket. The key that will unlock the door to new opportunities.

Yet at the same time, we do have a wonderful capacity to heal and to return to a life of vitality and richness, rather than carrying on in a debilitating version of reality that is both clouded and haunted by the past.

It's as if the brain isn't getting past first base. The right brain and the left brain are, if you will pardon the pun, at loggerheads with each other. As an individual recreates trauma in the mind, so the right brain gets triggered as if the traumatic event is happening in the present. And the left brain isn't functioning to capacity and is unable to bring its logical, objective analysis. Bessel van der Kolk writes that trauma sufferers can simply re-live the past as if it is in the here and now of the present moment, leaving them "furious, terrified, enraged, ashamed or frozen". And that's a really tough place to be. And that can be just as tough for their partners and families. (See Madeleine's story, chapter 33).

The argument goes that the rational brain cannot talk the emotional brain out of its reactive perceptions.

So how do we deal with this caged, pent-up energy?

Imagine we are living in a northern climate, where the environment is locked in by snow and ice all winter long. Then, one day, spring makes its first tentative entry into the scene. A spring thaw starts with a single drop.

Quite simply, we start to move.

The word "emotion" derives from the Latin "emovere" – which means to move. If we are frozen or stuck in rigidity, then we will not – and maybe cannot – move.

Think about those times when you have cried – or perhaps haven't. On many occasions, I have sat with clients who have been on the verge of tears. Perhaps ashamed or embarrassed to show tears, they have held themselves tightly in their own rigidity. I have silently wondered if they will yield to tears and, in a way, hoping they do so. Feelings derive from movement. Rigidity suppresses tears.

Movement allows the tears to flow, the facial muscles show grief, the breathing changes and vocal sobs are let out from the mouth. The release of crying is just one way to get moving. Nancy Kline affirms that crying actually makes us smarter.

Crying is perfectly natural. When we just sit with and listen to someone who is crying, without trying to fix them or smother them but just allow them to cry, to think, to talk, to think again, then they will often emerge with greater clarity – a greater movement of thoughts. Through their emotion, they have created their own motion.

Imagine the little boy who reached out to one or both of his parents, arms out and in tears, to cope with his upset feelings. And consider that parent standing, arms folded, responding with: "Big boys don't cry! Pull yourself together." Maybe on just one occasion, or perhaps repeated over time. Consequently, that emotion might turn back on itself, the boy might retroflect. He retains his emotions within his body. Done over time, he learns not to cry. To withhold and to suppress. And with a diminished perception of comfort and trust in others or with his external environment.

Movement can start with the slightest of motions – and it is important to get moving. Which brings us back to the brain moving so that the right and left brain don't remain in their personal lockdown.

Giulia Enders considers the possibility that the brain's purpose is to generate movement. She also invites us to consider where our sense of self is located. Where do you consider your sense of self to be? In your head? Or your heart? Or perhaps a combination of our brain and gut is crucial here. We will explore this concept, plus the three brains theory – in the head, heart and the gut – later in this book.

Let's get back to movement. Just watch a cat wake up from a nap. It will create movement. It will stretch itself upwards and then might stretch forwards and back. Only then does it begin to move.

And any athlete will tell you that exercise starts with stretches to prepare the body for more physical movement, to prepare the body for exercise. Both relaxation and considerable exercise can work wonders for stress. Stretch out your body to prepare your muscles for movement.

So relax, take a stretch – and get moving!

CHAPTER 10

Jane's story: waking up into a nightmare

I first met Jane at a European Mentoring and Coaching Council Research Conference in Holland in 2011. We were both making presentations, and we enjoyed talking together in the evening; our conversation facilitated through an attendant lip speaker.

As we chatted, we talked about coaching and Jane's two linked and traumatic experiences – losing her hearing and the impact that her deafness had upon her career, initially as a diplomat and more recently as a champion for those at society's margins.

That evening, I was struck both by Jane's *passion* for fairness and inclusion and her *compassion* for people with disadvantages. Jane went on to train formally with me as a coach and later returned to work with me on leading sessions on the application of body language in coaching.

I view Jane as one of those people who wants to see changes in society – and, simply, to help make the world a kinder and better place. Before you read her story, here are a few words from Jane on disability and discrimination:

The nature of disability

"Disability is non-elective personal circumstance. No disabled person would have chosen to be disabled. I, as an ex-professional orchestral musician, would certainly not have chosen to become deaf.

Disability is very personal."

Diversity good practice

*"Diversity good practice at work is to **acknowledge individuality**, with each person finding the best way for them to progress and develop. This is worked out with those who line manage and supervise the person."*

Waking up into a nightmare

Please give an overview of the traumatic event – what happened.

I worked for the British diplomatic service. I have been deaf since my early 20s and use human support at work. These are specialists called lip speakers who, silently, make English lip-readable.

I did a successful diplomatic posting to Poland for four years and had lip speakers there with me. It was a small team of between four and six people that rotated, and they usually did two weeks each.

At the same time, I did well-recognised additional work on disability rights and legislative reform on top of my role as the leader of a policy team. I spoke Polish confidently. I had learnt some basic Polish as a young adult just as I started to become deaf. I worked hard to improve my Polish using the Foreign and Commonwealth Office language training and used it every day on my posting.

In the final year of my posting in Poland, I applied for new roles overseas. This was highly competitive, and I had several interviews.

I was finally offered my 'dream job' of becoming a deputy ambassador – a great learning role for me as a middle to senior level manager. I got the job offer and was psychologically preparing myself for the new role.

But then a few weeks later, the HR department wrote to say that the job would be conditional on assessing my "reasonable adjustments" (i.e., the lip speakers) and that their analysis, using a new framework they had recently created, showed the cost of this would not be reasonable.

The trauma was prolonged. A mental health professional who assessed me later expressed the view that it was "the most extreme case of discrimination I have ever come across".

What is important when explaining this trauma is that no advice had been offered as to how I could negotiate my career within this framework. When I asked about this, the HR staff said that if they made suggestions or gave advice, this would be discriminatory!

So, in effect, I was being told that I could apply for absolutely any job I wished, and only then would they assess its 'reasonableness' (by which they meant cost – a frustratingly narrow approach which did not take account of any of the many other ways of assessing effectiveness at work).

This was an extremely isolating experience as I was the only one, as far as I know, of 14,000 staff globally who was being treated in this way. How could anyone else understand it? And the high cost of my support was basically being used against me – it felt as if I had deliberately caused this.

At no point was any specialist in disability, deafness or human rights offered. I was put at an extreme disadvantage (before even considering the damage physically, psychologically and emotionally this inflicted) and had to put forward my case as best I could, seeking support externally (on top of a demanding day job).

It felt that I had been chosen as what the jargon would describe as 'low-hanging fruit' – an easy target for 'cost savings' or 'efficiencies'. I was 'easy' because there was just one of me. At no point did any of those involved even pause to consider why I was the only one, and what the impact of treating me this way might have on the future diversity of the department.

For a period of several months, I would wake from what was usually a very brief sleep and temporarily forgot what was happening. When I fully woke up, it was to a living nightmare.

What, to me, was most harsh was that I was being asked to be a hypocrite. I had worked hard to promote the UK's equality legislative model – including disability rights. This was something I believe in deeply. Equality had been a strong personal value since childhood.

When Polish government contacts – with whom I had built successful relationships – found out about the posting being removed, they were astonished, as it flew in the face of everything we had discussed.

Just before it happened, the British Minister for Disabled People had visited his counterpart in Poland. The Polish minister praised the fact the UK had a diplomat who embodied its equality principles; the UK minister replied, saying that I was "an excellent example of the UK's equality rights in practice". In an international review of diversity in practice across the international network, I was the only officer referred to by name – for my work on disability rights.

This "excellent example" was basically told on the one hand that I had got the job on merit, but it was then withdrawn due to "reasonableness" – financial considerations.

You talked about going deaf in your early 20s, Jane. And I know you were a keen musician and played in an orchestra at the time. I'm only beginning to imagine how hard that was for you at that time. What impact did that have upon you?

Yes, that is right. Tinnitus (ringing and percussive sounds in both ears) started on my 24th birthday. Not a welcome gift! Some hearing loss then happened, gradually at first, then there was a dramatic loss.

The loss of music was, without doubt, the worst thing. I have described it as like having my soul ripped out. Losing ease of communication and social contact was the second worst. Not being able to access jokes and humour was especially painful, though I can now do this, mainly through finding the right support and friends who see it as natural that they should communicate accessibly.

I think it helped that I am an optimist, so never questioned that I would make my way in life and continue to work. Work and purpose were crucial.

What happened to your career as a diplomat after this happened? What did you do next?

I continued to work full-time for the FCO for about a year after the events I described. I was determined to do things on my terms.

I sued my employer and took part in an employment tribunal, followed by two appeal tribunals. I didn't win, despite bringing a strong case with backing from the Equality and Human Rights Commission (EHRC).

But importantly I got to air the issues and, also, live with myself. I would have felt like a hypocrite if I had allowed this level of what I perceive as blatant discrimination against me without challenging it.

Jane's claim against the FCO under the Disability Discrimination Act made national headlines. *The Independent* newspaper reported it like this:

Equality watchdogs have warned that disabled people face growing barriers in the workplace after a senior diplomat lost her discrimination claim against a Foreign Office refusal to send her abroad on the grounds her deafness made the posting too expensive.

Jane Cordell, 44, had a job offer to become Britain's deputy ambassador to Kazakhstan revoked by Whitehall after it was ruled that the £240,000 cost to the public of providing trained "lip speakers" could not be justified

But the Equality and Human Rights Commission (EHRC) said the ruling raised questions about whether it would be possible for Ms Cordell, who was praised for her previous work in Poland and earmarked for promotion, and others like her, to proceed as far as able-bodied people in their chosen careers.

In a copy of the ruling obtained by The Independent, *the tribunal said it accepted its ruling would place "some limitations" on the types of posting that Ms Cordell might obtain but added that the cost of funding the support needed to allow her to do her job was "simply unreasonable".*

The decision to withdraw her Kazakhstan job offer in January this year was based on legislation which obliges employers to make "reasonable adjustments", such as the funding of specialist equipment or assistance, to allow disabled staff to carry out their work.

A spokeswoman for the EHRC, which partly funded Ms Cordell's case, said: "The outcome is disappointing for Jane. It has left her career in a state of limbo as she has no clarity around what level of adjustments the FCO will fund – a decision which directly influences whether she can be posted abroad in the future. It is important that reasonable adjustments are provided to allow disabled people like Jane to realise their full potential….

The tribunal dismissed arguments that the cost of accommodating her deafness was being used unfairly to restrict her career when the FCO routinely pays out large sums for the private education of the children of diplomats posted abroad."

© Cahal Milmo/The Independent

Note

Keith writes: there you have it. The FCO provided lip speakers for Jane in Poland. Then it deemed it was not reasonable to fund the lip speakers in her new, higher-level role. But the FCO does pay for private education for diplomats' children. [Which, incidentally, would not have been necessary in Jane's case.]

A conversation with a recruitment expert who was a psychologist triggered an 'aha' moment in me. He said: "It doesn't sound as if the FCO is somewhere you can thrive."

That caused me to flip how I viewed my work and role. I moved away from thinking, "Can I contribute?" I knew I could and had demonstrated this clearly, but could I thrive in that environment?

I gave myself permission to work in an environment where I could thrive. An interesting role came up for a year at Action on Hearing Loss (then known as RNID), in Manchester, as head of a social enterprise team.

I took a secondment from the FCO then resigned on my 46th birthday (my gift to myself!) about 11 months later.

It was so interesting to work in a positive, accessible environment after the traumatic one I had left. I realise how context can define us. I regularly felt amazed that work could feel so "easeful" – and I felt very grateful for it. It was a wonderful transition job.

After a year, I was lucky to be invited to continue in the job but had taken a year to decide that I needed to have time for myself. I had thought for some time about trying to work for myself and had gained voluntary experience as a coach over the previous couple of years.

This seemed the right point to try. So in 2012, that was what I did, offering coaching and public speaking.

An opportunity to run a development programme for a local disability charity led me very fortuitously to meet Hormoz Ahmadzadeh at Result CIC, at that time a new social enterprise. The project went so well that he and his co-director invited me to join them. And that is my main role now as a director at Result CIC. It provides coaching and personal development training for people who feel marginalised. It draws on the lived experience of its associates, including us as directors.

Jane, it seems that your deafness was something that you had no choice but to accept, while you ultimately made a choice to leave your employer and take your working contribution elsewhere. How did these affect you cognitively, emotionally and physiologically?

That is true. You don't get a choice when you acquire a disability. So it develops your resilience: you have to get good at solving problems and negotiating the challenges which the disability causes – often issues about other people's behaviour and how they can make life more accessible for you.

The deafness did not affect me cognitively, as far as I am aware. If anything, it made me even more alert and even more eager to try to prepare and plan things to reduce the level of risk that I may miss information. I became more innovative! Physically/physiologically it made me tired – and still does. There is so much to negotiate to understand what people are saying.

What I did not realise at first was that my aural memory was considerable. Once I started to play viola again after several years' break, musical memory returned to me, and I would 'hear' things I had played and old songs in my head – which was incredible and so comforting.

Emotionally it was hard, though deafness also helped to clarify who really supported me (my friends, happy to say) and who didn't (the partner I was with at the time). Deafness is cruel because it makes conversation and social contact so much harder. And to feel better, what you need is… social contact. It is tempting to isolate yourself as a deaf person because being in a group can be a harsh reminder of what you are missing and can make you feel more left out.

In terms of the discrimination – I think the easiest thing is to attach a 'script' I used with Human Resources at the FCO before I had a meeting with them. I knew that facing them would be incredibly tough. So I decided to write what I wanted to say in advance, then I read it aloud to them. I give this text to students to whom I give a lecture annually at Leeds University Business School. It outlines the impact of the discrimination.

How can discrimination affect the individual employee? Jane's experience.

Extracts from a lecture presented by Jane in February 2020, describing the impact it had for her.

Note: *I will use the generic second person 'you' as I find this easier to relay, but this is my experience.*

a) **Physical impact**

The first effect of discrimination is **physical**. It is similar to someone in heavy boots kicking you in the ribs. You are winded, cannot breathe and you shallow-breathe for up to a couple of weeks afterwards. Then you have shock symptoms – you shake, shiver and feel sick.

This reaction repeats each time the discrimination is repeated or reinforced. [Such as in each email.]

The person being discriminated against then loses all appetite while the shock and stress symptoms take over. So you lose weight and feel literally 'fragile'. This means you are physically less well able to cope just at the point where due to the demands to somehow handle the discrimination, you need more, not fewer resources.

b) **Psychological impact**

After shock comes disbelief. "How can they do this?" A feeling of others dismissing and devaluing who you are and what you can do. There is then an intense anger and frustration which is exacerbated by language from the discriminators attempting to describe what you are feeling. In my case phrases such as 'very disappointed' and 'you are having a difficult time' are so saccharine and far from the reality they made the situation worse – if that was possible.

The control which the discriminatory behaviour exercises disturbs your sleep. This lack of sleep compounds the physical fragility started by the initial shock. The large burden of extra work created by handling the discrimination and, in my case, making my case for a job which I had been offered on merit, causes mental overload. Lack of sleep and over-stimulation compounds the fragility from the sick feeling and lack of appetite. Your stomach is almost permanently in knots. I regularly experienced vertigo and dizziness.

The way I described it to a concerned friend was the reverse of waking from a nightmare into reality: each morning you wake up and have to cope with the fact that your reality has become a nightmare.

The combination of physical and psychological effects could easily 'send a person under'. What helped me avoid this was anger that this could happen to other colleagues with disabilities who may well lack the confidence to handle it.

Another important psychological effect is isolation. I am the only person in the FCO to my knowledge who had competed for a job, got one, then had it removed on cost grounds related to my disability. Everyone who asked about this expressed disbelief and sympathy, but nobody could express empathy because nobody had been through it or could imagine what it was like.

As a prominently disabled person you have to work many times harder than your non-disabled colleagues to integrate into an almost entirely non-disabled workplace. Being treated in the way I have been can unravel much of that good work and cause a serious loss of personal confidence.

c) **Emotional impact**

Discrimination causes a deep sadness, verging on depression, a feeling of being fundamentally undermined, insulted and – it is not too strong a word – tortured. This obviously also had an impact on my husband and family who have had to watch me going through this.

You described optimism, work and purpose as being important for you. What else helped you at that time to move through these very challenging times?

I had some counselling after my mum (with whom I was incredibly close and who was also my best friend and like a sister in some ways) died in 2002, just less than a year after I had started at the FCO. I also had regular coaching when on a scheme for talented civil servants. Both these types of support helped me learn that I could control my thoughts (a bit like Cognitive Behavioural Therapy in the case of the counselling). I became an avid reader of self-help books – and still am.

Being asked to coach others on a scheme for disabled leaders (with Disability Rights UK) encouraged me to develop coaching skills myself. Supporting others in this very direct, personal way definitely helped me.

On the day of the final appeal tribunal, which we lost, I had arranged to coach a person with a significant learning disability who was also coping with the death of his father. There was no better way to put aside my own concerns, at least temporarily!

In addition to the formal roles you describe above, I know that you have chaired other social enterprises and charities, been a trustee for the Manchester Deaf Centre and been elected as a board member of the Arts Marketing Association. You have won awards for your work, been included in the Power 100 list of the UK's most influential people with a disability or long-term health condition and in 2018 made an Honorary Fellow of Liverpool John Moores University. You have also given evidence to the Parliamentary Work and Pensions Select Committee for reviews centred on employment and disability. How important has it been for you to channel your energy in this way, linking it to your values and your purpose?

It has been very important. But I did not set out specifically to be involved in these areas. What I did was try to be clear about how I wanted to use my experience and skills positively. Then gradually, these roles and opportunities found me. I was asked to try for various governance roles by people who seemed to see my potential.

The roles meant that I could use the earlier traumatic experiences to benefit others, even if indirectly. And like an alternative powerful route to continue the work I started in Poland (on disability equality).

How do you practice self-care?

By learning from experience and observation.

It was only a couple of years after the discrimination and tribunals, when life became quieter and more easeful, that I realised one day there was an absence of pain – no headache, no blocked-up feeling, no back ache, no digestive tension, no exhaustion, no mental stress.

I remember walking locally and asking myself, "What's different?" Then I suddenly realised – the presence of absence – it had gone! It was a valuable moment and I vowed to learn from it. So I started trying to work out how to feel better, what I needed to do in terms of types of exercise, eating, sleeping and, importantly, the type of work and activity I engaged in.

I only discovered some time after they happened, for example, that two of the physical symptoms I experienced during the discrimination had official names.

First, I started to find it hard to swallow sometimes when I was eating – I would feel as if I was going to choke. This was usually when I was at work at the FCO (which is significant). It was scary. It's called dysphagia and can, apparently, sometimes be caused by stress.

The second was dissociation – which is a condition where you can suddenly feel separated from your own body – you view yourself from the outside in a critical way – you 'see yourself' from a distance. That happened regularly and was really disorienting and frightening.

When I later thought about this, I wondered if it happened because there was a public 'me' who was taking the government to court – a campaigner and activist who was, reluctantly, in the news, and a private me who felt incredibly vulnerable. I thought that the dissociation was almost a manifestation of that.

I am still learning about what helps me most, and I like the process of learning. I recently came across the concept of being an 'empath' – someone who tends to absorb others' energy automatically and feel others' feelings. This helped explain several things to me.

There can be a reluctance to exercise self-care if it is associated with 'selfishness'. I realised many years ago that unless you practise self-care, you cannot give the best support to others.

Finally, Jane, what advice would you give to others? Whether they have a disability, are marginalised, or are recovering from their personal trauma?

Each person has to find the way that works for them. Each of us is different. Trauma forces us to know ourselves deeply, sometimes in painful and very unwelcome ways. But we get to know ourselves and often have to ask questions of ourselves that we would not do otherwise. That said I think there are a couple of things it can be useful to do, depending on your own situation of course.

It is worth standing back from the situation to look at where you had (or have) responsibility. Make sure you are crystal clear about the boundaries between your and others' responsibility for the situation or event. Then appreciate that your role may be smaller than you think and try to drop any guilt-based emotional baggage which was linked to the negative event and you subconsciously assuming too much responsibility.

I would also recommend that you check where you do have power and control and then focus on those areas, maximising their positive impact. Think about the choices there are, not the ones which you feel may have been removed. This moves you into a psychologically and emotionally much calmer and stronger place, and you will be able to take better decisions for yourself as a result.

The other thing which I would advise is to ask people you trust for support. Nobody needs to go through a trauma alone, even if you feel you are the only one on the planet going through the experience. Ask, and most of the time, people will help if they can.

Finally, be aware of what you are learning, very painful though it may be. What 'muscles' are you developing, for example, your resilience and a healthy perspective? Acknowledge these things and fold them into your personal store of skills. You may be surprised how well they will serve you in future.

Part 3

Acceptance

Accepting what has happened is a crucial early step in recovering from traumatic and difficult experiences.

Yet it can be a challenging process, as you allow yourself to come to terms fully with the events from the past and explore and acknowledge the impact they had for you – and are continuing to have for you in the here and now.

Preceding acceptance are resistant behaviours such as:

- Denial – denying that it has impacted you.
- Minimising – kidding yourself that it wasn't too bad.
- Deflecting – stating that others are in a worse place than you.
- Repression – banning or holding back unacceptable or painful memories.
- Rationalising – explaining away difficult emotional situations.

In the long run, such behaviours impede progress. They tend to keep you stuck, which isn't going to enable you to move forwards.

Enter acceptance, enter awareness. Accepting what has happened is a vital here-and-now opportunity for you to come to terms with your past, acknowledge what has happened and start to grow your awareness.

Chapter 11

Accept yourself for who you are and for what happened to you

Terrible things happened, but they are history.

The benefits of acceptance can't really be underestimated. Accepting that you are you. Accepting that what has happened has happened. Accepting the impact that it has had upon you. An aide of former US president Richard Nixon famously pointed out that you can't squeeze the toothpaste back into the tube. The toothpaste is out. It's up to you what you're going to do with it.

Traumatic and challenging experiences happen. You can beat yourself up and tear yourself apart looking back over your life, but this doesn't really help. It's too easy to have regrets. To think back and say to yourself, "If only I..." or "Why did it happen to me..." or "I should have..." and so on.

You can't change the past. But there is good news. The past has passed. It is over. I am inviting you to put aside any sense of "what might have been" and simply accept what happened – and then allow yourself to be more fully in the here-and-now of the present.

Your past events have brought you to where you are today. And it's the legacy of those past events that can continue to be corrosive today. What is happening for you right now and the impact it is having upon you.

Acceptance is fundamental to the change process. Once you have accepted and brought into your awareness the past, you can then more fully explore new ways. It's the equivalent of a new way of

Edward Bear not only coming down the stairs but also opening the front door beyond the bottom of the stairs and exploring and enjoying life outside in new and energising ways.

Let's return to the theme of toothpaste for a moment. I don't know about you, but I remember going to work one day, only for a kind work colleague to let me know that there were the remains of dried, white toothpaste plastered across my cheek.

And you know what? That's life. Stuff happens. Life's messy at times. We all have our toothpaste moments. And we can always wipe the toothpaste off.

Once we're aware of the toothpaste, we can do something about it. Acceptance and awareness: two crucial aspects of the developmental and healing journey. We will explore both of these crucial themes as we explore the theme of acceptance.

CHAPTER 12

The past has passed

Trauma's place in the past.

One view of the purpose of studying history is that that we can learn from our past mistakes. And it seems that sometimes we do – and, to our cost, sometimes we don't. The 2020 pandemic has been compared on many occasions with the last great pandemic – the 1918 Spanish flu. I'm not sure how many lessons we learnt. Perhaps in the comfort of our 21st-century lifestyle, many people didn't think it could happen again. It seemed as if we had been in denial.

On a personal level, think about your relationship with the past. Are you liberated by your past? Constrained by your past? Stuck in your past? Have you let go of your past? One of the effects of difficult and traumatic experiences is that they can, if unchecked, allow the past to maintain an extraordinary grip over the psyche. We can go through things in our mind, over and over again…

- What happened?
- Why did it happen?
- If I hadn't gone out that night…?
- Why did I stay married so long?
- I wish I had…
- If only I had listened to…
- He should have…
- I should have…

These are some of the thoughts that might haunt us. Perhaps for a day or two. Or a week or two. Or much longer…

Yet the past is over; it cannot be brought back or replayed.

As a teenager, I remember worrying about something one day. My father noticed this and asked me what I was worrying about exactly a week ago. I couldn't remember. His point was that worries are thoughts – and thoughts can come and go. We can let them go. I remember repeating this exercise with a friend who seemed to be worrying a lot. She then told me not only everything she was worried about today but was also worried about a week ago. No two people are the same! It was a useful exercise to try out. You can try it out on yourself too. Just what exactly were you concerned or worried about this time last week?

It's easy to assume that the past is the past, but how often have you paused to consider your relationship with your past? As indicated above, have you let it go, or does it keep a hold on you? Or somewhere between? Every one of us will have our own unique relationship with the past.

Imagine a group of people (usually in their 40s to 60s) going away for a 1980s weekend. The event might typically focus on a couple of evenings dancing to 80s music, as Abba and Wham songs are belted out over the dancefloor to bring back memories of days gone by. And many enthusiasts will have dressed appropriately to re-live the memories of that era.

But are they celebrating the past or living in the past? There is a big difference.

Celebrating the past allows the person to step back into the past and then come back into the present moment. Yet living in the past is a personal realm of duality. It is a jarring dichotomy of past and present. There is the reality of a 'safe' and 'normal' present – perhaps as simple as completing a straightforward task. Then there is the reality of the past memories – as if being hijacked and disappearing down a dark hole of overwhelming, agonising trauma. These memories can be triggered as easily as flicking on a light switch. For a good friend, something as simple as washing the dishes after dinner. Although the friend was in a safe place, he could so easily be triggered by past memories that flooded him in the here and now of the present moment.

There is a world of difference between stepping into and out of the past, re-living younger days, and being held captive by the past, as illustrated below in Jenny's story.

Case study

Jenny's story

Jenny had a reasonably successful career as an administration manager in a business. She always showed up for coaching sessions immaculately dressed. Smart blue business suit, shiny shoes seemingly ready for military inspection, precise haircut, manicured hands. Everything was in order, nothing out of place. Lots of self-control, but there was seemingly no spontaneity, and her team members were becoming very frustrated. Everything was by the book, with, apparently, no scope for creativity.

It appeared that Jenny was very controlled in everything she did. Her appearance, her demeanour in the coaching, her behaviours at work. Within the coaching sessions, she was very controlled too.

It wasn't until we had held a few sessions that she revealed that her father had suddenly and dramatically committed suicide when she was 13. Jenny had discovered his body. As she told me this, tears were forming around her eyes. But they never fully materialised. It was as if Jenny had become frozen at that time. Her coping strategy with it as an adult was to exercise very high levels of control. No surprises, no spontaneity. Apart from her husband, she had never told anyone what happened when she was 13. She had never been offered help and had never sought help.

The first 13 years of her life had been spent as a child, growing up. For the subsequent 30 years, she was caught within the net of the traumatic experience, coping with it through high levels of personal and environmental control. One third of her life as a child; two thirds of her life as a highly controlled adult. I don't know why her father committed suicide, and I'm not here to judge. But I have often since wondered whether he might have changed his mind, given the awful legacy he would pass on to his teenage daughter.

For those with such traumatic experiences, its grip can be so tight. It is a case of loosening that grip, little by little. And whatever your personal unfinished business from the past, you can start to ease it away, step by step.

Janina Fisher proposes that individuals "are ready to heal the injuries caused by the trauma" when they are sufficiently present in the here and now and can deal with the usual swings and roundabouts of normal living.

Whatever has happened to you in your past, you are here. You are an ingenious survivor.

We will shortly move into the present, but before we do so, let's take a brief look at the critical topic of unfinished business and its effect on people who have had unresolved traumatic or difficult experiences.

CHAPTER 13

Unfinished business from the past

You can never swim through the same river twice. You are different today to how you were yesterday.

Most of us have unfinished business from the past. We have seen how traumatic and difficult experiences from the past can be described on a continuum, from the mild through the substantial to the severe.

At one end of the trauma scale, we might just feel frustrated or uncomfortable. These are mild effects. At the other, Phil Joyce and Charlotte Sills describe how PTSD can lead to crippling, repetitive symptoms. At these extremes, the authors contend that the trauma sufferer may be left with emotional or somatic [in the body] symptoms. In such experiences, being and becoming more aware of emotions, being and becoming more aware of your felt sense becomes so important. Perhaps the trauma was overwhelming, happened a long time ago, or experienced at such a young age that it disappeared out of conscious awareness. Yet the individual can be triggered by events today that are experienced physiologically but which remain beyond awareness. The process of transference 'transfers' our past experiences into the present moment.

Working through unfinished business allows the individual to move closer towards closure. Keeping things out of conscious awareness ties up a lot of energy that could be utilised more usefully elsewhere.

By considering the scale of the impact created by the trauma or difficult event, it is possible to see what support and resources might help the individual to close the unfinished business.

If it is mild, then the individual will often recover in a short period of time. Talking it through with family or friends, coupled with internal processes, might suffice.

If it is more substantial, then talking things through with a counsellor might be necessary. Or the individual might also work with a coach. As Joyce and Sills write, it's the "support, emotional expression or closure" that enables an individual to move forward from the past.

Specialist therapy is required at the more severe end of the spectrum. The therapist works carefully and at a pace that is safe for the client and does not re-traumatise the client.

Raising awareness, letting go of the past and transitioning to the new can take time – particularly as the 'old' responses have been coping strategies which, repeated over time, have felt 'safe'. The journey then is letting go and recreating, moving towards a newer sense of self.

This can be very powerful work, which is when therapy becomes so valuable. And the traumatic memories can be whole body work too, inhabiting both the body and the mind.

Yet as well as benefitting from external support, it is within the individual's power to do many things – and to 'be' in ways that will help them move from the past into the present to create a better future.

And that's the aim – to deal with and bring to closure unfinished business, to be better able to move forwards.

After all, by and large, we like happy endings, don't we? Those romantic stories when the hero and heroine end up happy ever after. Or the action films when good triumphs over evil and we can get up from our sofas and make a cup of tea, knowing the world is safe again.

The pandemic has been a bit different though – repeated waves, a succession of new normals. The uncertainty of not knowing when or how it's going to end or how many more friends or relations (or even ourselves) might succumb to its deadly effects.

Unfinished business can be understood through the following example. Back in the 1930s, Bluma Zeigarnik made a study of waiters in a café. Research revealed that waiters had a better recollection of unpaid orders over those that had been paid up. It felt unfinished – therefore lingered in the memory as something of a tension. It's distinct from completed tasks – those times when we forget about something that is neatly finished, allowing us to move on. Imagine you've got a dripping tap. Until it gets fixed, it's unfinished. Calling in the plumber resolves the problem. Only then is there closure.

A lot of things happen to us as we go through life. We build up a vast reservoir of life experiences. Some of these we recall with fondness, others with sadness or perhaps anger. Some feel finished, others less so. Just look through your family photograph albums and see what memories and emotions you notice as you rekindle those thoughts and feelings from years ago.

Understanding and coming to terms with unfinished business from the past can yield a great deal of satisfaction. This is particularly helpful if you have had experiences that might still be located and locked within you today.

For those who have suffered traumatic experiences, this could be particularly impactful. Think of this in terms of breathing. Watch sportsmen and women getting ready for action. You might see them breathe in and pump their chests, preparing themselves for combat. They may be in aggressive mode. Or at the other extreme, you may encounter people who are empty chested, as if their chests have deflated and collapsed. Petruska Clarkson contrasts these positions as aggressiveness and resignation. This is different from healthy breathing – as practised in yoga. In such breathing there is a rhythm and a flow; it is healthy. But with rigidity – when the chest is aggressively puffed out or resignedly collapsed, then there is tension, there is rigidity. It is sometimes called body armouring. And the chest is just one example. Many people do not realise that some of their muscles are continuously tense – or armoured.

These can leave people stuck. They can lead to repeating patterns that don't yield satisfactory outcomes. It's often heard in their language. It is as if recurring patterns occur. Let's look at Harry's story.

Case study

How Harry's unfinished business kept popping up

While Harry was growing up as a child, one of the messages he heard from his father was "beware of the bogeyman".

I asked what impact it had on him.

"My dad didn't mean any harm," said Harry, "but it was one of those messages that I kept hearing. Even as a young child. For many years growing up, I was always on the lookout for the bogeyman, I guess. I never seemed to fully achieve. Or afraid that somebody would take something away from me."

"Can you give me an example?"

"Yes, I was a pretty good runner at school and would usually be in the top 10 in races against other schools. One day, there was a road relay in a nearby town against 20 or 30 other schools. Each team had six runners who each ran a leg of just under two miles. We came third as a team, and I was really pleased because I ran the fastest time of the day – of all runners. It was the only time I achieved that."

"And the bogeyman?"

"At the prize-giving later in the afternoon, the sports teacher from the host school was giving out the awards for the fastest runners of the day. As he gave out the medals, he said: "Modesty prevents me from saying who actually ran the fastest time of the day, but the fastest time goes to Harry…."

"Can you explain?"

"Yes, he was a runner himself and had raced round the course too."

"You really noticed that, didn't you?"

"Yes, it took something away from running the fastest lap. The only time it happened."

It was one of those events that had really struck a chord with Harry. What was significant was that he really noticed it, it triggered a reaction in him. Another person might not even have heard it, or heard it in a different context, and not been bothered about it. But it impacted Harry, even though the teacher was an adult, while all the runners were in their teens.

Listening to him, not judging, helped to validate his experience. We then went on to explore how the imaginary bogeyman might be affecting him in his adult life, in his work.

Harry went on to share that he found negotiations difficult.

"I find it difficult to trust people. I'm worried they are going to engineer the deal for themselves in a bad way. And I've had a pattern of seemingly upsetting or provoking people who have then attacked me personally."

"To what degree is this 'real' or your interpretation?"

"It's difficult to say really, but I do notice them."

"I'm wondering if your mind is almost waiting for the bogeyman to pop up at any time."

"I remember once introducing a new graduate scheme at work. It was my responsibility – and it worked very well. When it had completed, we had a graduation ceremony, which was a great success. I was very proud of it."

"Go on."

"Near the end, the CEO – who had handed out the awards – came up to me and said two things. Firstly, he congratulated me, then he asked how we could do it better next year."

"How did that leave you?"

"Flattened – a bit dismissive. It took the wind out of my sails."

We then explored the links between the two events and how they might be connected. We also explored feelings of (not) being good enough – but largely focused on something being taken away. We spent some time unpicking the motives behind the CEO's message. Perhaps the pattern of a fast-paced, directive leader who possessed only a limited array of leadership/motivational skills.

Reframing the situation in this way enabled Harry to reflect back on what had happened, looking at it through a different lens.

What was noticeable was what Harry noticed. What really stood out for him.

His pattern of people and situations in life that became his version of 'reality'. What it was that made these experiences significant for him. And equally significant in a manner that another person would simply not experience in the same way. A useful tool is to notice what you notice.

How we experience life: figure and background

What is figural for you in life? What patterns do you notice that recur in your experiences? Joining the slowest queue in the supermarket or post office? Bossy, arrogant people who interfere with your work? The beautiful sounds of birds singing in the wild? Never finishing work on time and always staying late? Notice those things in your life that become figural – that really stand out for you. Or to put it simply, notice what you notice.

Right now, as you are reading this book, the words are, I hope, most figural. But imagine that your phone rings or buzzes. That might catch your attention (it becomes more figural), especially if you are expecting an important call. It might become even more figural if, for example, you are being harassed by an ex-partner who still keeps in touch. The figure is what becomes prominent within your attention. It emerges from the background – known as the ground – which is available to us all.

To understand what is meant by ground, imagine you are in a business meeting with 11 other people. The 'ground' is the room and everything therein. The people are sitting around a large, rectangular, wooden table. The chairs are blue, the carpet is grey. Windows are located on one side of the room. A large, black TV screen is attached to a wall. Coffees and teas are in the corner. The air conditioning is on, and the air is slightly cool. Stacks of papers are on the table. That ground is available to everyone. But it might be experienced very differently by the 11 individuals in that room.

The first person might be impatient to get the meeting started and finished because he has 'better' things to do.

The second person might be flicking through messages on her phone, anxiously waiting to receive the latest monthly sales figures.

The third person is retiring in two months' time and is relaxed and doesn't really care too much about the meeting.

The fourth person has just been appointed to this group and is nervously looking around, wanting to make a suitable impression. She feels slightly chilly and anxious.

The fifth person had an argument with her husband that morning and wonders if he has been unfaithful.

The sixth person chairs the meeting and wants to make sure it runs on time and is effective.

The seventh person finds these meetings tiresome and only attends begrudgingly.

The eighth person is making a presentation and is checking through his presentation slides.

The ninth person hates meetings. As a child, she was criticised by the teacher in front of the whole class. It was traumatic. She feels exposed, not wanting to appear stupid.

The tenth person suffers from claustrophobia and finds the room a bit stuffy and intimidating. He is feeling panicky.

The eleventh person is keen on promotion and wants to impress the chair.

So just imagine how each individual will arrange the 'ground' in a personal way. Where is their attention? What is figural for them? How aware are they of the here-and-now in the room? Each person will have their own version of 'reality'. Different people will be aware of different things. The 11 realities will be a mixture of what is in the room, but also a potpourri of how they mentally arrange their ground, based upon their historical experiences, beliefs, values, anxieties, patterns – and this is often how they will construct their reality. And for each of them, there will be significant differences. I wonder how many of the 11 will be fully present rather than somewhere inside their mental constructs in their heads.

Activity

Notice your ground and see what becomes figural.

Staying where you are, notice your ground. Allow yourself to become aware of your surroundings. This is called undirected awareness, when you just allow yourself to observe and notice. What becomes figural for you? Once you have noticed something for some time, allow your attention to focus on something else. After a few minutes, jot down some notes about each of these.

What I noticed	Notes
I saw…	
I heard…	
I felt…	
I smelt…	
I tasted…	

You experience the world through your senses, and this exercise on awareness invites you to notice how you are experiencing the environment around you – the 'ground'. Now cast your mind back to two recent events. One of which was a pleasant experience, one of which was unpleasant. And then complete the table below.

What I noticed	Pleasant experience	Unpleasant experience
I saw…		
I heard…		
I felt…		
I smelt…		
I tasted…		

Finally, what patterns, if any, do you notice? Use the space below for your reflections.

Allowing your mind to consider the ground – as in the exercise – will help you to move away from 'inside your head' to focus your attention on what is 'out there'. This allows you to become more aware of the environment. By becoming more aware in this way, you are turning down your internal self-talk and allowing yourself to become more aware of – and in tune with – the environment (the ground) you are in. Incidentally, planting both feet on the ground (whether sitting or standing) is a useful grounding activity. Consequently, you will be more present in the business meeting described earlier. Indeed, you will become more aware wherever you show up in life.

And if you have experience of trauma, these types of exercises can be particularly helpful to allow yourself to be more open, deploy your energy more constructively and be more focused on the matter at hand.

Chapter 14

You're OK, I'm OK. We're OK. Okay!

I accept you. You accept me.

I have a very simple belief system with my clients – and with people in general. With clients, I'm OK and they're OK. Or if I am with you, I'm OK and you're OK.

I like that philosophy. It underpins all my work. We might have had tough times, we might make mistakes, but we're still OK.

I have found it to be a good philosophy for coaching. It allows the client and me to chat on an even footing.

- I might disagree with you, but you're OK. You might disagree with me, but I'm OK.
- I might not share your values, but you're OK. You might not share my values, but I'm OK.
- I might not agree with your behaviour, but you're OK. You might not agree with my behaviour, but I'm OK.
- I might not agree with your beliefs, but you're OK. You might not agree with my beliefs, but I'm OK.

To sum it up, I'm OK with you and you're OK with me.

When coaching, I work to an appropriate code of conduct, follow the law and am aware of extreme occasions when it might become necessary to disclose details of the conversations – but that's absolutely right for coaches, counsellors and therapists.

So, a key learning point for us all is to acknowledge to ourselves that we are OK.

Rooted in a psychological approach called transactional analysis (TA), the proposition is that you are either in an 'OK' or 'not OK' life position.

Consider the wife and husband who have had an argument early in the morning before heading off separately for work. It started off on a seemingly trivial incident but then grew. Eventually they both stormed off, their unfinished disagreement lingering with them all day. According to the TA model, they would be in one of four life positions:

Life position	In two words	Summary
I'm OK – You're OK	**Win (+) : Win (+)**	Both parties are OK with each other. They might disagree but accept and respect differences.
I'm not OK – You're OK	**Lose (-) : Win (+)**	I'm in the wrong and you're in the right
I'm OK – You're not OK	**Win (+) : Lose (-)**	I'm right and you're wrong
I'm not OK – You're not OK	**Lose (-) : Lose (-)**	I'm in the wrong and you're in the wrong

So which box might the arguing couple be in?

They're clearly not in the *win:win* situation. They both stormed off, issue unresolved.

I'm not sure they are in the *lose:win* situation – certainly to start with. The fact that they were confrontational suggested they were both coming from a position of being in the right. The person who puts themselves in the 'I'm not OK' box thinks/feels they are in the wrong and the other person is in the right. (However, as the day wears on, one or both might migrate into this box.)

They might both be in the *win:lose* position, that the other is in the wrong, which could lead to an animated homecoming later in the day.

Finally, they might also be in the *lose:lose* position. In this case, both parties may be angry and think the other is in the wrong. However, on reflection, each might realise that they have gone over the top and said things that they didn't mean to say. For example, they shouted something in the heat of the moment, which they now feel bad about. They are still angry with their partner but also regret their words and possibly their actions.

Life's like this – in different situations and contexts, you may recall occasions when you have been in each of the four boxes.

It takes a turn for the worse if you regularly find yourself habitually in one of the "not OK" quadrants. Those relationships when the pattern of communication, like *Groundhog Day*, is repeated over and over again. Consider the "I'm not OK : you're OK" position – there can be a regular underdog/top dog outcome. People who have been in abusive relationships may recognise this quickly. Key to this is noticing the body language and hearing the words that are used. Read through the table below for some dire dialogues.

- **I'm OK : You're not OK:**

   "You shouldn't have spent that much money on a dress."

   I'm not OK response:

   "I'm sorry, dear, I'll take it back."

- **I'm OK : You're not OK:**

"You really ought to cut the grass this weekend. You said you would do it."

I'm not OK response:

"I will try to do it later. I didn't mean to let you down. I'll do it after I've cleaned the windows. Enjoy your time in the spa."

It's a sad fact of life that far too many people go through life feeling 'not OK' about themselves or perhaps 'not OK' about aspects of their character of appearance.

The child who has suffered abuse growing up is an example. The 'not OK' position can become, through repetition, their life's prison. If they were to write their own school report, it might read 'could do better'. Sadly, this life position is surprisingly widespread. And it is a pretty disheartening way to go through life. You might notice it with people who work long hours every day. They think they could do better, so simply work harder. You might have heard of the phrase 'imposter syndrome'. In a single sentence, it can be heard as 'When are they going to find out I'm not really up to this?' It's not unusual for highly successful people in highly paid jobs to feel an imposter, despite their apparent 'successes'.

It is also not uncommon to see a difference in someone's professional and personal personas. Highly successful in a work capacity, but much more uncertain personally. They might be the type of person who champions others' needs and goes into battle for others but don't recognise or attend to their personal needs. They might find it difficult to say 'no', for example. These people might be acutely aware of their responsibilities, but not in touch with their rights as an individual.

Below is a list of rights that you have. Take a look through these and tick the ones that you personally recognise within yourself. These are your rights as a human being.

You have the right to...	Tick these if you believe these apply to you...
Turn down an invitation from another person to feel 'not OK' or bad	
Have feelings and opinions and express them freely and appropriately	
Have clear personal boundaries	
Broaden or narrow your personal boundaries	
Be successful	
Make mistakes	
Make decisions – and then cope with the consequences	
Attend to and use your intuition/gut feeling	
Ask for what you want or prefer (Do recognise the other person's right to say 'no' as well)	
Privacy	
Say no – without feeling the need to justify or feel guilty	
Confront	
Change your mind	
Be flexible	
Feel OK even when your knowledge and understanding aren't total	
Change and become assertive	
Be a carer towards others (not a rescuer)	
Feel pleased with yourself	
Be happy	
Feel confident	

And remember that you have the right to have rights. You may want to add to this list. As long as you do not seek to abuse the rights of others, then it is an assertive right.

Now that you have read through the list, what might be your development areas, if any?

Once you have completed the list, there's one thing that I recommend you to do.

When you reflect upon yourself, look at this through a position of compassion and self-care.

I cannot overstate the importance of this. Please do not look at yourself through a filter of being overly critical. (Too many people are their own strongest critics. We can be constructively critical and still feel OK, which is different.)

None of us has all the answers, but we're OK. None of us is perfect, but we're OK. Welcome to the human race!

Activity

Your development areas

Having read through the list above, are there any areas that you notice are particularly relevant to you? Perhaps as strengths or opportunities for growth. Note them down, together with your reflections around each of these points. Reflect on this without judgement – make sure you complete this exercise while being in the 'I'm OK' box!

Strengths: Occasions when I am 'OK'	Opportunities for growth: Occasions when I am 'not OK'

When you have completed this, just notice which of these become prominent.

Finally, choose one development area and answer the questions below.

How would I need to think and feel to move from the 'not OK' to the 'OK' box?
What is my first/next step on my journey to the 'OK' box?

Chapter 15

Feel your feelings for self-awareness

Feelings are giving you valuable data. Notice them.

Some people talk about feelings as either being 'positive' or 'negative'. I often prefer not to do that – to avoid placing judgement on feelings. Feelings are just feelings. Some might argue that anger is a negative emotion and that it is not acceptable to feel anger or to behave in an angry manner.

I recall someone once who had this philosophy. She was adamant that she didn't become angry about issues. As she spoke, and as I probed her with questions about anger, she became more and more animated, and her neck became suffused with a dramatic shade of red. She would not countenance anger in herself, but what I noticed was somebody who was angry. And this vignette suggests many things. Anger is a basic emotion; she lacked emotional self-awareness about her anger; she seemed unable to recognise or describe the anger; she was in denial about her anger; she was carrying inner tensions around the topic; she was attempting to suppress her anger; the suppression was inhibiting her ability to become more fully present; she had internalised a belief system around anger. And so on. Of course, these are only my hypotheses, but I noticed there was a lot going on.

And if you consider anger as a negative emotion, then consider my anger for a moment. I feel angry about the scale of domestic abuse in this country. I feel angry when one person abuses another. I am not suppressing my angry feelings here. I don't consider anger in this context to be negative. I am owning the feeling of anger and describing it. I believe I am justified in expressing these feelings. I do consider, however, there is an important distinction between controlled anger and uncontrolled anger. That's different; that's when the red mist descends, and an individual loses control.

Notice your feelings for a moment.

- Where are specific feelings located in your body?
- What might your body be communicating with you? [Are you noticing it?]
- Do feelings create thoughts, or do feelings result from thoughts?
- Notice your energy around specific feelings. Are these energising or draining?
- Feelings can be contradictory [Guilty pleasures.]
- Feelings can often be repressed – but at what cost?

If you are in touch with your feelings, you are likely to be more energised. If you are unable to recognise or express your feelings, then they may leave you tired or depressed – and can lead to anxiety. Suppressed feelings – particularly from childhood – can lead to feelings of numbness and emptiness.

Two of the things I've noticed in coaching is how people experience their feelings.

- Firstly, they can sometimes seem overwhelmed.
- Secondly, a difficulty in distinguishing feelings from thoughts – and then a challenge in describing those feelings.

When people tell me their stories in coaching sessions, they often do so in a very animated way. They might talk about a topic that has disturbed them, and I ask them to scale the feeling on a 1 to 10 score, when 1 is low and 10 is high. They will often rate it as an 8 or 9. Next, I ask them to recall a truly awful moment in their life – without me needing to know about it. I invite them to rate that event as a 10 – it is the worst. I then ask them to reflect further upon the 8 or 9 rating they have given to their current topic and ask them how they would scale it now. Often it drops to between 3 and 6. Through this process, I am inviting them to scale their feelings differently and not to be so overwhelmed with the topic under discussion. You can try this scaling approach on yourself and your feelings.

I also invite them to describe the feeling in their own words. After all, the phrase "I'm angry" is open to lots of interpretations – are they just irritated or really mad about something?

There are also many occasions when I ask someone how they feel about something, and they answer with a thought. Here's an example:

Keith: "How are you feeling about your weight right now?"

Client: "That I should go to the gym."

It's an example of asking a question about feelings, but the client replies with a thought. There are emotions contained within the reply, and these relate to going to the gym. And not particularly energised emotions either. If you can recognise this within yourself, then I suggest you can do two things.

Firstly, distinguish your thoughts from your feelings.

Secondly, allow yourself to notice, feel and become aware of your feelings.

Four of the fundamental feelings we experience are joy, sadness, anger and fear. You might have heard them described in terms of questions – what makes you sad, mad, glad or afraid? These are very broad headings. When you read through these, you will notice different, more specific descriptions. It's a useful exercise in terms of reflecting upon your emotional vocabulary. If you find yourself unable to describe your emotions specifically, then you might find the lists below helpful. As you read through these, notice what happens to your feelings and energy levels.

Words associated with sadness

Defeated	Dejected	Depressed	Despair
Desperate	Despondent	Devastated	Disappear (desire to)
Disappointed	Discouraged	Dismayed	Embarrassed
Guilty	Helpless	Hopeless	Hurt
Ignored	Inadequate	Incompetent	Inferior
Inhibited	Insecure	Isolated	Lonely
Melancholy	Miserable	Misunderstood	Muddled
Needy	Pessimistic	Pity	Preoccupied
Pressured	Regretful	Rejected	Remorseful
Self-conscious	Shy	Sorry	Stupid
Tired	Trapped	Troubled	Unappreciated
Unattractive	Uncertain	Uncomfortable	Unfulfilled
Useless	Victimised	Violated	Vulnerable
Weary	Worried		

Words associated with anger

Annoyed	Bitter	Contemptuous	Disgruntlement
Disgusted	Displeased	Distrustful	Enraged
Exasperated	Frustrated	Furious	Hateful
Humiliated	Huff (in a)	Hurt	Ignored
Impatient	Indignation	Insulted	Irritated
Miffed	Outraged	Overwhelmed	Provoked
Raging	Resentful	Stubborn	Touchy
Unappreciated	Uneasy	Vengeful	

Words associated with joy

Affectionate	Alive	Amused	Anticipation
Beautiful	Brave	Buzzing	Calm
Capable	Carefree	Caring	Cheerful
Cherished	Comfortable	Competent	Concerned
Confident	Contentment	Courage	Curious
Delight	Desire	Eager	Ecstatic
Energised	Euphoric	Excited	Feeling good (self)
Forgiving	Friendly	Fulfilled	Generous
Giving	Gleeful	Good	Gratitude
Happy	Hopeful	Humorous	Joyful
Lovable	Passionate	Peaceful	Playful
Pleased	Proud	Quiet	Relaxed
Relieved	Respected	Safe	Supportive
Sympathetic	Tender	Thankful	Thrilled
Trusted	Understanding	Understood	Unique
Valuable	Warm	Witty	Wonderful
Worthwhile	Youthful		

Words associated with fear

Afraid	Apprehensive	Ashamed	Desperate
Devastated	Dread	Fearful	Frantic
Indecisive	Helpless	Hopeless	Horrified
Insecure	Overwhelmed	Panicked	Pressured
Scared	Self-destructive	Self-loathing	Terrified
Threatened	Timid	Trapped	Uncertain
Uncomfortable	Victimised	Violated	Vulnerable
Worried			

Feelings and the body

Edmund Bourne writes about how these feelings show up in the body as tight muscles. He suggests tensions can be a common symptom of "chronically withheld feelings". He writes that anger and frustration can be suppressed by the tightening within the back of the neck and shoulders; grief and sadness by tightening muscles in the chest and around the eyes; and fear through tightening in the stomach/diaphragm area.

Activity

Your feelings

Reflect upon the feelings described above and apply them to yourself. Think about events in your life over the last few days. Work through the rows in the table below. Consider how you can bring more focus to these feelings. And notice how much more precise these descriptors can be. Identify four individual feelings – one from each section – and complete the table below.

Basic feeling	The specific feeling you notice	What you notice about it
Sadness		
Anger		
Joy		
Fear		

Next, relax and pay attention to your body. Where do you notice the feeling in your body?

Basic feeling	The specific feelings you notice	Where you notice this in your body
Sadness		
Anger		
Joy		
Fear		

Finally, use the space below to note down your reflections from this exercise.

Chapter 16

Connecting with your body

There is no one else quite like you in the world. Accept and cherish who you are and what you bring.

No one has to be traumatised to become self-conscious of their body. In the celebrity era, much attention is paid to looks. Yet as Anita Roddick famously stated, there are just eight out of three billion women who look like supermodels.

In our 'comparison' society, people can allow themselves to be pressured to look a certain way and to keep up with fashion trends as one season gives way to the next.

It's all too easy to tie up a lot of energy:

- ...trying to keep up with the "more praised" sibling
- ...trying to keep up with the neighbours
- ...trying to keep up with the supermodels
- ...trying to ward off those wrinkles.

I have purposely used the word trying four times. It becomes very trying and consequently tiring. So much trying to be or look like something occupies so much energy. It becomes another façade we present to the world.

How about a bit of self-acceptance instead? How about stop trying to be someone else and become more self-accepting? And self-loving? Beauty comes from the inside. Think about your relationship with your body. Does it feel integrated and accepted? Or are there some parts that you wish you could change, or perhaps you have allowed yourself to become alienated from? And considering long-standing trauma, perhaps there are parts from which you feel disconnected.

People's concerns can be around many different things. Too many wrinkles, small feet, big feet, large nose, stocky thighs, large breasts, small penis, small breasts, large penis, furry eyebrows, hair that's too straight, hair that disappeared years ago, gappy teeth, small hands, too small, too heavy, thin lips... the list goes on.

Of course, many of us want to look and feel 'good', to walk with confidence in the world and to strengthen our sense of self. Perhaps we can distinguish between a desire for healthy changes and less healthy ones.

You can start by considering how you might integrate more – or all – aspects of your body and mind. Reframe your relationship with yourself not only holistically – how you see yourself as a whole – but also from your specific body parts. It's your body that carries you through life, so it's wise to appreciate it. (As yet there is no Body B.)

None of us is perfect; that's what makes us human. Consider those people you know who might want to project 'perfection'. I know many people who are frustrated with partners who want to be perceived as 'perfect'. I'm not sure I would want to spend all day and every day with someone who projects perfection. My message is simple. Learn to love yourself, warts and all. Okay, so maybe you want to address those warts, but allow yourself to do this from a position of choice and healthy self-regard.

Do consider yourself as a whole. It brings to mind the statement that "the whole is greater than the sum of its parts". At the end of the day, we are composed of cells and tissues, but we are much greater and more complex than these. So, if we choose to fret all day about our wrinkles (thereby frowning and making them worse) or angst that we don't have the 'body beautiful', aren't we missing the point?

Hold your bigger picture.

- You are you.
- You are a unique individual.
- There is no one else on this planet quite like you.
- Cherish yourself.
- You bring your special uniqueness to the world.

Chapter 17

Symptoms of trauma: learn to respond rather than react

Switch off the autopilot and choose how to 'be' in the moment.

There are many diverse symptoms of traumatic experiences, such as anxiety, depression, avoidance, panic attacks, flashbacks, insomnia and so on. These derive from the tensions held both in the body and mind. Peter Levine (1997) contends that "each of us has had a traumatic experience" during our lives and that it is so commonplace that most of us aren't aware of its presence. And if we don't recognise its presence, then we're very unlikely to be aware of the full impact it has on our daily lives.

It's useful to distinguish between reacting and responding:

React: When you go to the doctor, and the doctor taps your knee to test your reflexes, your knee will automatically move. This is a reaction. There is an automatic reaction to the trigger. You cannot help it.

Respond: By becoming (more) aware of the trigger – and the impact it has upon you – you allow yourself the luxury of the choice. You can choose to respond rather than react.

Raising awareness in yourself is such an important starting point in your journey. Once you are aware of your triggers and your reactions, then you begin to have the opportunity to change. If you are not aware, then you will simply repeat the same patterns of behaviour. A liberating outcome of raised awareness is that it leads to greater choices – you have the opportunity to empower yourself.

Bringing these triggers more and more into your consciousness gives you greater opportunity to gain more control over them, rather than them controlling you.

Learning to respond rather than react creates a wonderful opportunity for you to move forward, to shift your position. Events will happen in your life that you have no control over. What you do have control over, however, is how you choose to respond to them. Learning this can take time, and it is important to take the first steps to gain traction and hence movement.

Case study

Keith's salutary coaching lesson

I was coaching Lucy, a 54-year-old woman who had been talking through a particular challenge she was facing. It was one of those moments when I lost some concentration and said, rather clumsily: "You can only do your best."

I somewhat regretted my words the moment they came out of my mouth.

"That's what my mother used to say," reacted Lucy, her irritation evident. She was not happy.

Curiously, the next 10 minutes of the coaching allowed us to explore her reaction.

My ill-conceived words had, interestingly, opened up a new discussion that ultimately helped both Lucy and me. Those words had triggered this reaction in her, which had been within her for over 40 years.

It was a timely reminder to me about how important words can be. My choice of words had taken her back to being nine years old again. They had remained within her unresolved for decades. They tapped into her vulnerability. Curiously, although they had been clumsy, these words opened new opportunities for exploration.

Something else that it helps to be aware of as a coach is my body language. When I am concentrating and seeking to understand a client, there can be a slight furrowing of my brows, which resembles a frown. On a few occasions, clients have noticed this as a frown and assumed I am judging them. I have learnt the following:

- My words or gestures can provoke a reaction – even the slightest frown.
- The client has a vulnerability that might emerge from my words or gestures (frown). In the examples above, the clients had a susceptibility to feeling judged.

From these examples, it can be seen that a single sentence, word, look or gesture can trigger a strong reaction in the client. At its extreme, it can provoke a traumatic reaction. It has the potential to recreate the original traumatic event. My words triggered the client. It took her back to her childhood. Consider an abusive relationship and remember this. A single word, look or movement can trigger a traumatic reaction. That reflects the level of control and power that can be exerted by one person over another.

Life's like that. For Lucy, the unfinished business from decades earlier. It is valuable to remember that all our relationships are coloured by our earlier relationships and experiences. And we often have a stronger memory of our 'bad' experiences rather than our 'good' ones. Consider a day at work when you have completed 10 tasks. Nine went well, but one didn't have the outcome you desired. When you get home, which one of the 10 is most figural in your mind? It's usually the one that didn't go as planned. Maybe you are being triggered by the one task that went less well. Allow yourself to choose to recognise the nine that went well, learn from the tenth and move on.

Learning to respond rather than react enables us to create more choices. And it's our choices which say so much about us – much more than our capabilities.

Choose to respond, choose to show who you truly are. Allow yourself to be who and how you want to be in your life.

Chapter 18

From dissociating to connecting

Becoming integrated in mind and body.

To understand dissociation, it helps to go to the experts, so here are two descriptors. Firstly, from the American Psychological Association (APA), and secondly, from the UK's National Health Service (NHS).

The APA describes dissociation on its website:

> "A defense mechanism in which conflicting impulses are kept apart or threatening ideas and feelings are separated from the rest of the psyche."

The NHS website describes dissociative orders in this way:

> **"Dissociative disorders are a range of conditions that can cause physical and psychological problems.**
> Some dissociative disorders are very shortlived, perhaps following a traumatic life event, and resolve on their own over a matter of weeks or months. Others can last much longer.

> **Symptoms of a dissociative disorder**
> Dissociation is a way the mind copes with too much stress.
> People who dissociate may feel disconnected from themselves and the world around them.
> Periods of dissociation can last for a relatively short time (hours or days) or for much longer (weeks or months).
> It can sometimes last for years, but usually if a person has other dissociative disorders.

Many people with a dissociative disorder have had a traumatic event during childhood.

They may dissociate and avoid dealing with it as a way of coping with it."

The NHS highlights both a traumatic life event and a traumatic event during childhood. (There can also be repeated trauma, such as with an abusive parent.) The consequences indicated above may last from a few hours to much longer – even to the extent of becoming internalised for a lifetime (and even role-modelled on to subsequent generations).

In such instances it may lead to a dissociative disorder. The NHS website states:

"Switching off from reality is a normal defence mechanism that helps the person cope during a traumatic time.

It's a form of denial, as if 'this is not happening to me'.

It becomes dysfunctional when the environment is no longer traumatic, but the person still acts and lives as if it is, and has not dealt with or processed the event."

The pandemic triggered many traumatic and challenging events. Consider this. How is death experienced? Is it traumatic? Perhaps it is a release. If someone has lived a long life and dies peacefully of old age, then we can look back on their lives and appreciate the richness of their life.

Death in other ways may well be experienced as traumatic. A sudden or unexpected passing, perhaps the victim of crime or a motor vehicle accident, or a sudden death, or a terrorist attack. Or the circumstances of too many deaths during the pandemic: its suddenness; inability to visit dying loved ones; no chance to say goodbye; the cruel reality of socially distanced funerals. Then there are the health professionals who have witnessed so many people dying, day after day after day in appalling circumstances. And after that, the consequences for mental health – for the bereaved families and for the many exhausted nurses and doctors. One way or another, the pandemic has affected us all.

The felt effects of the pandemic might be experienced as trauma, overlaying pre-existing traumatic experiences. These may be strikingly different experiences, or variations on a theme. In this case, it may lead to complex post-traumatic stress disorder (CPTSD). In such cases, the individual has experienced different traumatic episodes.

It can be a lot for the brain to handle. Getting on with daily life while at the same time experiencing ongoing traumatic effects. I wonder how big that disassociated divide is – a crack? Significant gap? Chasm? And much of this going on subconsciously, not infrequently in a state of hazy and vague awareness but felt consciously through tension and easily triggered reactions.

It's why the self-awareness journey is so vital. If you are aware of something, you have the opportunity to change. If you are unaware, then you are unlikely to change. Unawareness is like a blind spot in the mirror. Awareness brings more into your consciousness.

Then the journey becomes that of bridging the gap. Connecting, integrating, building bridges. And those bridges, those connections, really help when they are in place.

Janina Fisher describes such gaps as "internal self-alienation" and explains it as the "disconnected" left brain focusing on daily life, while the right brain "remains in survival mode, braced for danger". Or, as the APA stated previously, the feelings separated from the rest of the psyche.

And that is what can happen. One half coping with daily living, the other like a rabbit in the headlights, wanting to find escape or, as she writes, "too ashamed to do anything but submit".

That leads to a tense state of affairs, really, as the individual attempts to navigate day-to-day life. Dealing with this survival mode while also carrying on as best as possible as the competent and capable manager/leader/wife/husband/father/mother – or whatever roles the individual's life position asks from them.

What a struggle this can be! Imagine the amount of energy that is tied up in this exhausting daily ride with its inner tensions. It's such a tough place to be. It's a pretty exhausting way of living a life. Challenges – perceived as threats – have the habit of popping up at any time. How to cope when presenting at a meeting? Or having an intense discussion with your partner? Or wanting to be a firm but fair parent? Or a boss whose behaviours – or frowns – trigger memories of a critical or abusive parent?

It can be difficult to get on with a "normal life" while dealing with all this running around in the head. And a lot of the time, just not understanding what is really going on and why these patterns just repeat, repeat and repeat.

Imagine the scenario of the physically or emotionally battered wife who wants to leave her abusive husband but can't. And her friends who witness her plight, but then become frustrated with her for not leaving. It can be so difficult to leave, to crawl out from under the weighty rock of years of submission and an abusive and manipulative partner. To integrate both sides of the brain and to avoid the internal hijacks. Perhaps she has frozen, perhaps she has flopped, or perhaps she has fawned – soothing the abuser to avoid more anguish.

But there is good news. There is the opportunity to heal. To go from dissociation to association, from un-integration to integration, from dismember to remember. It is the journey to wholeness.

You can write new stories for your life, feel safe and feel close in new relationships. Yes, you really can. The following are facts:

- You can build more integrated, internal connections.
- You can turn down dramatically the heat of those old thinking, feeling and physiological patterns.
- You can create new patterns for yourself – and reinforce your new patterns. You can say "I'm OK".
- You can push back.
- You can punch back.
- You can fight back when you choose, walk away when you choose.
- You have the choice to choose.
- You can pick your battles.
- You can say "no" without feeling the need to justify your reasons. Or yourself.
- You can see those red flags and choose to cross the road.
- You can feel whole within yourself.
- You can become more of who you want to be and who you want to become.
- You can accept invitations and decline invitations.
- You can set your agenda.
- You are in control.
- You can live your life the way you want to.
- You can choose when to give and when to take.
- You can feel whole. You are whole.
- You can be who you want to be.
- You can choose to live the way you want to live.

And remember this.

You have the key in your pocket.

Activity

It's helpful to be alert to the words and phrases we apply to ourselves in our everyday language. Below are a number of phrases that you might have heard yourself saying. Perhaps such phrases are used infrequently, or sometimes more regularly. Have you heard yourself saying these?

- "I'm not feeling myself today."
- "I'm really in two minds about this."
- "I'm a bit all over the place."
- "I'm feeling torn."
- "I'm feeling a bit out of sorts."
- "I feel as if I'm falling apart."

Do any of these sound familiar? It helps to be aware of the impact that such self-talk can have on the psyche. And perhaps these can be replaced with different, kinder phrases. If you have recently heard yourself saying one of these phrases, then I invite you to do the following.

1. Consider how you can empower yourself.
2. Re-write the statement in a more positive light.

In the table below are two examples of this. Use the row in the bottom of the table to write down a phrase you might have spoken, and then complete the row.

Phrase	Empower yourself	Alternative phrase
"I'm really in two minds about this."	I am perfectly capable of making a decision. I will do so when the time is right for me. It's a complex decision, with pros and cons.	"I can and will make the decision when I am ready."
"I'm a bit all over the place with my parenting."	I can only be in one place at a time, and my feet are on the ground. There are many things to consider.	"I'm a good enough parent, and that makes me a very human role model for my children."

We have a wonderful capacity to heal. Just as we might have 'dis-membered', so we can 're-member'; as we might have alienated, we can join; as we might have detached, so we can attach; as we might think we lost the plot, so we can write new stories; as we might have disintegrated, so we can re-integrate; as we might have separated, so we can become whole. We can come back to ourselves.

So if there is disconnection, then start the journey to connection.

1. Start to re-connect.
2. Continue to integrate.
3. Allow yourself to be fully joined up.

All we're doing is bringing ourselves back together.

Chapter 19

Nurture and enrich the inner game of your life

Turn down the volume of your inner critic, and tune into your inner wisdom.

There's an old saying in tennis that the opponent inside one's head is more formidable than the opponent on the other side of the net. The saying could be translated into other sports too. And it could be extended into work and many other areas of life. Who might be the opponent in your head, for example, that gets in your way at work, or perhaps in relationships?

Back in the 1970s, a man called Tim Gallwey reinvented tennis coaching.

In his book *The Inner Game of Tennis*, he described how traditional tennis coaches – himself included – would instruct their players on what to do. Coaches would tell players how to hold the racket, where to put their feet and so on. Crucially, subjected to such critical and intrusive instruction, he noticed that the players, instead of improving their performance, often made more errors. Gallwey also observed their ability – or inability – to compete effectively. Perhaps they might freeze at match point or be one of those players who trained well but couldn't convert that into competitive success.

His conclusion was that the coach's traditional approach of telling players what to do actually hindered, rather than helped, the players. It was causing (psychological) interference. Hearing critical or instructive words would create a psychological trigger that led to involuntary bodily reactions. Increased bodily tension inevitably impacted personal performance.

At which point he decided to adopt a different approach – and one that is based upon a different adage – keep your eye on the ball.

Rather than shout out instructions, he asked the player to become more aware.

- What did the player notice about how the ball was coming onto their racket?
- What did the player notice about their serve that might have made the ball go too far and being called 'out'?

His open questioning approach invited the player to take more control. It gave ownership and accountability to the player. This approach empowered the player and led to greater focus and calmness within her game, which led to higher performance.

Gallwey noted players came to him to "fix" a part of their game. They disempowered themselves by handing the responsibility for their performance to the coach. Yet by developing greater trust in themselves, he noticed their performances improved – and with seeming effortlessness.

He developed this into a theory of Self 1 and Self 2.

Self 1 gives the judgements – the critical voice that wants to take control. What Gallwey described as the 'know-it-all' that had internalised all the messages taken in from the outside world.

Self 2 is the player's ability to learn naturally. Self 2 is where the fundamental, innate power and potential reside, and all too often it can be overridden by Self 1 – the voice in the head.

These are the wrong way round – this is the tail wagging the dog. This is the inner (critical) voice in the head which interferes with and has the power to sabotage performance.

Gallwey described this through an equation:

Performance = potential – interference.

I have a simple view in life. None of us is performing at our full potential. What gets in the way is interference, or Self 1 – those internalised critical messages that have the debilitating effect of limiting performance. This inner voice comes from a place of faulty self-image. This distorts perception, interferes with the player's ability to perform, and leads to mistakes – sometimes called unforced errors in tennis. Which, of course, brings the player back to mistakenly confirm – and mistakenly prove to herself – her distorted self-image. The result, over time, is a vicious cycle.

Just imagine the impact on performance for the 19-year-old aspiring tennis player with the following voices in her head as she goes on to the court:

- Parent: you've always been a choker.
- Coach: remember not to choke at the big moments.

It brings to mind again the famous Henry Ford quote. "If you think you can, you're right. If you think you can't, you're right." The one thing that is sure to be on her mind is choking.

To raise performance, Gallwey proposed three factors:

1. Non-judgemental awareness.
2. Trust in your inner self (Self 2).
3. Keep choice with the choice-maker.

There's that word again – awareness. It is a case of turning down the volume of the inner critic (all the way to mute if you can) and then trust yourself. How much do you trust yourself? Or how much do you allow yourself to be swayed by others, perhaps against your instinct? And then what choices do you make? Do you go along with others? Or do you make choices that simply follow a predictable pattern

– the choices you always make. In other words, are you actually making a choice – or deceiving yourself into thinking you are? What might be stopping you from allowing yourself to try a different path or head off in a different direction – one that you fully own? One that is a real choice?

Let's explore the origins and development of the 'inner critic'. Consider someone who has suffered some degree of criticism growing up.

- "You're the sporty one. Your sister's the bright one."
- "You'll never be good enough to play professionally."
- "You're a stupid child."
- "It's your fault, you shouldn't have…"

There are countless thousands of these. Maybe we recovered from these, maybe we didn't. But it doesn't take much imagination to consider the devastating amount of interference and/or judgementalism that can arise from a traumatic episode.

- "I'll never be any good at that."
- "I can't serve."
- "I can't paint."
- "I'm worthless."
- "I hate myself."
- "I'm useless."

These are corrosive self-messages and, as seen earlier, the distorted self-image leads ultimately to distorted results – which just reinforce and recycle the distorted self-image.

And consider those occasions when that criticism has been repeated time and time again. Or has been dished out to the young person after she lost a sports match or *'failed* to perform' in an area of activity. Perhaps afterwards, she sat on the back seat of the car as dad picked apart her performance. Trapped in the car until she could get home and escape. It could be experienced with some degree of trauma, especially if delivered harshly and/or repeatedly. And, of course, the player in the back of the car could internalise these messages in different ways. To confirm "I'm not good enough", or, of course, to drive them on: "I'll prove them wrong" (fight response) or just to get out: "I'm quitting" (flight response).

Gallwey's approach is based upon the fact human potential and performance can be released and enhanced in a very kind, accepting and respectful manner. Criticism, through judgement, really doesn't help very much – especially when that becomes an internalised voice in the head.

A good place to start is by being kind(er) on yourself. Remember, every time you criticise yourself in this way, it is like pouring petrol on a fire.

Activity: completing sentences

Allow yourself to complete the following sentences:

When I accept myself non-judgementally, I…	
When I trust myself, I…	
When I make the choices that feel right for me, I…	

What do you notice, having completed the sentences above?

Chapter 20

Live in your body, safely

You've only got one body. Look after it.

Every year in the UK, any car over three years old must have an annual MOT test. That involves getting a certificate. It will be checked for roadworthiness and safety. It will be tested for lights, electrical wiring, battery; windscreen, wipers, washers; steering; suspension; seatbelts; fuel system, body, vehicle, general items; seats; boot, tailgate; towbar; exhaust system and emissions; doors; mirrors; horn; brakes; tyres, wheels; bonnet and registration plate.

Here are two questions for you.

- How often do you check for your 'roadworthiness' or safety?
- When did you last check your 'roadworthiness'?

Or do you just carry on regardless until, like the car, you one day reach a juddering halt in the middle of the road?

To recap, cars on the road that are over three years old must have a roadworthiness certificate. It's a bit different when it comes to people. In England, the NHS offers a free health check for adults between 40 and 74. The NHS also offers a mental health 'assessment' which is not age-dependent.

Of course, a car certificate protects not only you and your passengers in the car but also other people you might pass on your journey, such as other vehicles or pedestrians.

Here's another question for you. How safe do you feel:

- With others, perhaps those you work with?
- With those at home?
- Within your own body?

Consider it as the external world and the internal world. The external world is 'out there', while the inner world is what is going on within your body and mind. This can be tough if you are coping with the effects of trauma. Bessel van der Kolk writes that: "...traumatized people chronically feel unsafe in their bodies."

In this position of re-lived trauma, it's possible for people to be unaware of their gut feelings, to experience numbness, to remain dissociated, to hold tensions in different parts of their bodies. Cast your mind back to Gallwey's interference in the last chapter. Struggling with the internal messages and not being able to access their Self 2, their inner strengths.

Think about it as the car. A broken mirror limits or blocks your vision; a worn tyre risks skidding; broken washers mean that you cannot see clearly ahead; a faulty seatbelt puts you at risk. The car becomes unsafe. But for the body, the warning signs are often ignored. The traumatised person can become bewildered, confused and ashamed – and become fearful of fear itself.

It's when therapeutic interventions become so valuable. Therapy establishes a safe place. And safe places are so important.

Yet what can we do to care for ourselves, to begin to allow ourselves to more fully experience our bodies? To re-establish or strengthen our body-mind connections. To allow ourselves to inhabit our bodies more. These are powerful themes to consider and explore.

Case study

Keith and the podiatrist. The podiatrist's story

The podiatrist was attending to a problem with my foot. I asked her how busy she was – which led to a wider discussion on people and how they look after their feet.

"You would be amazed," she said, "about how people look after – or rather don't – their feet. For example, I see many women who are extremely glamourous and well-presented. They look great, have immaculate hair, wonderful hands and nails – but their feet are in an awful condition. Because they are out of sight, many people do not look after them."

We went on to discuss the importance of our feet – after all, they take our weight and are our primary means of getting about. But notice the neglect. And then what happens as a consequence. It's an example of how we can separate ourselves off from different parts of our body.

When someone is unfortunate enough to sprain a wrist, it gets strapping or is put in a sling to heal. If the wrist is broken, then it gets put into plaster for a few weeks, followed by physiotherapy to strengthen the muscles that have wasted during the immobilisation period. Interestingly, after physiotherapy, some people come back stronger.

But what about body-mind connections? Physical slings and plasters aren't appropriate, probably because it's not visible to fix. Doctors might sign a patient off work for stress, prescribe medication, or even recommend some counselling (usually a fixed number of sessions). But what about something more precise and focused? The equivalent of a sling or a plaster? How best can we support ourselves to enable us to heal? Perhaps we can use our imagination to create our own slings and plasters to allow ourselves to heal. The start point is to attend to yourself. Give consideration to all parts of your body too.

Keith's story

My discussion during treatment with the podiatrist, above, led me to notice more about my skin – and some patterns over the years. Dry skin and athlete's foot (which is definitely un-athletic, by the way) are just two examples. As a schoolboy, I remember the day I forgot my plimsolls for the gym lesson. Anxious at the consequences (usually a detention), I borrowed a friend's and ended up with over 20 verrucae. Another one popped up recently. A couple of years ago, I had a basal cell carcinoma removed. All of these have rational explanations, but I wonder if there is a pattern here. The trauma I experienced many years ago was, after all, invasive.

And think about your skin, which protects you, cushions you from bumps and regulates your temperature. It is your protective barrier with the outside world. And it's crucial for sensations when you have contact with the world outside you. Like other body organs, your skin is very clever. Not only is it your largest sensory organ, but the outer layer, the epidermis, renews itself approximately every 27 days.

It makes sense to take care of your skin. According to nursingtimes. net, approximately half of the UK population will experience a skin condition in any given year. I mentioned earlier about giving consideration to different parts of your body. Often, it's easier to think about your back, or your hands, or your head than it is your skin. Attend to your skin too. After all, it's what holds you together. Well, for another 27 days until it renews itself.

Activity: notice your body

Allow yourself to relax and just to notice your body. You can do this in two ways.

1. **How you are in the here and now**
    Notice your body, both externally and internally, in the here and now. What do you notice?

2. Your history, your patterns

Think about your body over the years. Are there any particular areas or patterns that come to mind? Again, simply notice these.

[ ]

3. Reflections

From (1) and (2) above, what are your reflections, and what might you do to bring your body – and its parts – more into your awareness?

[ ]

Summary

Write down what you notice from 1-3, above.

[ ]

Chapter 21

Emotional intelligence – using your head and your heart

Everything starts with awareness.

Daniel Goleman's book *Emotional Intelligence* appeared in the 1990s and created a fresh framework for describing a person's emotional intelligence – their ability to cope with life on a daily basis.

Emotional intelligence (EI) invites you to access and then apply your thoughts and feelings. It is head and heart combined.

It is what you think and feel about something, and how you can use your thoughts and emotions to steer you through life more effectively. Imagine I am in some sort of relationship with you (which could be either personal or professional). Imagine within our relationship or living/work context we have a problem to resolve. It is what I think and feel about it, what you think and feel about it and how we might bring our thoughts and feelings together to resolve the issue to our mutual satisfaction.

- The rational person might say: "Let's look at this logically."
- The emotional person might say: "My heart rules my head" or "I wear my heart on my sleeve."

The rational approach leads to the problem being addressed purely logically. The emotional approach leads to the decision being reached through emotions. By contrast, the emotionally intelligent approach leads to the decision being made through a combination of both logic and emotions. Attending to our emotions can be very helpful in decision-making. Our emotions provide us with important data.

Traditionally, a person's IQ has been accepted as a solid measure of their intelligence. And no CV seems to be complete without a summary of qualifications, highest and most recent first.

Yet EI – or Emotional Quotient (EQ) – invites us to shift our perspectives. Proponents of emotional intelligence have claimed that our capacity to develop our self-awareness, handle our emotions, build relationships with others and manage our relationships are strong predictors of success in the world of work. There are people with huge IQs but who have low relatability with others. And in our more modern, digital world of work, our get-on-with-others-ability is recognised as extremely valuable.

Goleman's approach to EI positioned it into four main areas underpinned by motivation.

Self-awareness: being aware of our thoughts and emotions; being able to notice and describe emotions.

Self-management: the ability to manage thoughts and emotions. (If you are angry, being able to handle that feeling of anger, rather than letting the red mist descend.)

Social or relationship awareness: being aware of the dynamics of relationships; to notice the cues, to "read the room".

Social or relationship management: the capacity to handle relationships effectively. Capabilities such as assertiveness, empathy, building rapport, and the ability to handle differences.

And supporting these four areas is personal motivation; the energy that we bring to ourselves and our interactions in a broad range of contexts.

Consider the person who "storms" out of a business meeting in a fit of rage or hurt. [Not the wisest thing to do because, sooner or later, that individual will need to return if they are to remain part of the group.] For a moment, put aside who was right or wrong, the nature of the discussion and so on.

He left the meeting because he was *unable to manage the relationship* in that particular moment. He got triggered. The fact that he was unable to manage the relationship stemmed from a lack of awareness of the dynamics therein – *he lacked relationship awareness*. Then scroll it back to self-management. Clearly, he *was unable to manage himself* because he walked out. And he was unable to manage himself because he became triggered, because someone or something happened that pressed his buttons. And that comes down to *his lack of self-awareness*. He couldn't manage the relationship because he was unable to manage himself. He couldn't manage himself because he lacked self-awareness. Self-awareness is crucial.

Everything starts with awareness.

Developing your self-awareness is fundamental to how you go about enhancing your daily life and applying your coping strategies. Growing your self-awareness is the golden thread that runs through this book. What you think, how you feel, what your instinct says and what you are going to do with this.

The more self-aware you become, the greater the opportunity you have to create change within yourself. This has the opportunity to lessen the time you spend on autopilot, leading to you becoming triggered. Awareness can enable you to recognise those occasions when others press your hot buttons.

Consider these triggers – and your awareness – through the following metaphor.

Be like a fish when swimming through a river frequented by anglers. Bait-covered hooks will be cast into the water. Make a choice. Don't swallow the bait. Don't get caught on the hook. Hooks are painful and will do you not good at all. Don't rise to the bait. And if it's not a good river to swim in, then swim further up or downstream to a safer, more peaceful location. Find a protected, rocky outcrop that anglers can't get to. Getting triggered is like being caught on a hook – except that the hook is your own.

To return to the theme of hot buttons above, these are sometimes described as 'crumple' buttons. Those moments when a person can psychologically and emotionally implode from a particular situation or someone else's words or behaviours. Cars have designated crumple zones. A structural safety feature that protects you if your car should crash. It stops you from getting crumpled. A very good defence is to have your own air bag that inflates very quickly to protect you. Perhaps you can imagine yourself equipped with your personal air bag – ready to be inflated to protect you.

As self-awareness is crucial to growing your emotional intelligence, then a great place to start is with self-acceptance.

None of us is perfect. For many years I have used the Reuven Bar-On emotional intelligence profiling tool – the EQ-i. It provides a series of measures for individuals to self-assess their EQ. One of those measures is self-regard. One of the patterns I have noticed is that if an individual has low self-regard, then it can undermine so many other aspects of their daily functioning.

If we can accept ourselves, then we can have healthy self-regard. That ability to look at ourselves and say, "I'm OK with who I am."

Remember this. Be OK with who you are.

Chapter 22

What is your gut saying?

Attend to your gut.

Have you ever paused to consider how deeply the stomach is ingrained within everyday language?

You might not be able to stomach someone's behaviours or find it difficult to stomach an unresolved issue at work or home. One person might have butterflies in her stomach while the next one is contemplating his navel. You might not have the stomach for a certain task, or recently experienced an event that turned your stomach. Or your stomach might be grumbling. You might have gut feelings, gut reactions or gut instincts. You might even be gutted. You might want to get something out of your system. Going upwards, you might feel obliged to swallow your disappointment, or hear something that makes you want to throw up. You might need to chew something over, or even spit it out. Or you might have to bust a gut to finish some work that will otherwise go belly up. Going downwards, you might have had the crap scared out of you.

When you read these sayings about the stomach, notice how much emotion is conveyed in those everyday phrases. The feelings emerging from our guts are pretty powerful!

We may be able to recognise those feelings we describe as 'gut feel' or 'gut instinct'. I remember a coaching session in which I invited the client to consider all three:

- What do you think about…?
- How are you feeling about…?
- What is your gut instinct about…?

Interestingly, it was in the last of these (and I followed them sequentially, as shown) that movement (pardon the pun) emerged in the client. It was as if she connected with herself through becoming aware of her gut instinct.

Our gut instinct is so important – there is so much connective activity between the gut and the brain – and attending to these messages is so valuable. Notice your gut feelings. They can keep you safe and alert you to dangers. It's not always easy to understand that gut feeling – it operates at a deeper, more instinctive level. How many times have you heard yourself – or others – saying: "I wish I'd trusted my gut."

Attend to your gut. What might it be communicating with you? Julia's story is interesting.

Case study

Julia's story

Julia had been married with two teenage children, one of whom had left home for university, while the second was in her final year at school.

"I had long been unhappy in my marriage," said Julia. "My eldest daughter had left for London a couple of years earlier, and my younger daughter was going to join her. It filled me with foreboding."

My husband was very controlling around the house. The home had to be very clean when he came home after a day at work, otherwise he would become angry with all of us. We nicknamed him 'the examiner' as he checked all the rooms. There was trouble if they weren't clean...

He controlled the finances very tightly and had been keen for me to give up working. But I enjoyed my job. I worked as an IT trainer, and it gave me the opportunity to get out of the house and be myself. I dreaded the prospect of stopping work."

As we continued the discussion, Julia described her toilet patterns.

"I'm one of those people who could only go to the loo in my home," she said. "I used to tense up anywhere else, and it would only be when I was home that I felt relaxed enough to use the toilet.

Then it changed. As I became more aware of the controlling nature of my husband – with me, the children, finances and so on, it went into reverse. I noticed I relaxed when I was training in a company's offices or in a hotel. I rarely went to the loo at home but, in a relaxed setting, would have no problem at all. It was as if there had been a complete switch."

Some time later, Julia left her husband and now pays more attention to her gut.

"One of the things I notice now is my gut instinct – it is as if it has a mind of its own. I have started relationships again, but it is difficult for my gut to relax. Psychologically I feel relaxed, but my gut is still tensing up into knots. So now I pay more attention to it. It's telling me that my body is still on a journey towards relaxing."

Consider Julie, above. Consider the messages going on within her body flowing between gut and mind. The act of simply noticing has increased her awareness of her gut, her body. This starts to give her choice moving forwards.

Allow yourself to trust your gut, trust your instinct.

Activity

Firstly, notice your gut feelings – perhaps you can recall these from the past, or you can feel them now. What do you notice about them?

More specifically, pay attention to your gut right now. What might it be communicating with you? Simply notice, rather than become analytical.

What I am noticing about my gut

What it might be communicating with me

Chapter 23

Survive your way

Discover your way to healing: do what works for you.

I remember watching a video on YouTube. A cat had dragged a seemingly dead duck into its owner's home and left it on the floor. The cat's owners had filmed the scene as the duck lay lifeless. I thought it was a strange film to record but continued to watch. The cat walked away. The duck remained motionless for some time before suddenly flapping its wings, squawking into action and flying desperately out of the cat's reach to try and escape.

Nature has this wonderful capacity for defence. The bird or animal plays dead. Its energy is both shut down and ready to be released. It might have been injured by its attacker but lies motionless. Once free and away from its perpetrator, it shakes itself down and carries on with its life.

Case study

Lea's story

Lea's home life with her two cats was put under siege by a feral cat stalking the neighbourhood. The tom cat would take any opportunity to sneak into her house, eat any food left out and fight with her domesticated cats. Her cats paid a price. Neither would venture into the garden alone and one would pace relentlessly up and down in a heightened state of stress. Lea was also paying the price of the vet's bills for the injuries to her cats and had to keep all windows shut. Eventually the feral cat was humanely trapped and rehomed. Within a couple of days, her cats had returned to their former relaxed state. The difference was remarkable.

Humans seem less equipped to behave and recover than do the cats and duck described above. We explored the concept of dissociation earlier. The website Mind (2020) states that trauma can cause dissociation because of the way people respond to threat – often through fight or flight. And if these are not possible – which is often the case with young children – you might freeze or flop.

When someone freezes, the body and mind are numbed. You might feel that you cannot move – you are paralysed. With the flop response you become the rag doll. Your brain's thinking processes are shut off. You flop. You submit. Mind states: "our instinctive reactions to threat are the basis of dissociative experiences."

While people freeze or flop and dissociate, the duck and the cats recover. Humans are different. Peter Levine writes that "the supercharged energy locked in the nervous system is imprisoned by the emotions of fear and terror."

The recovery response does not take place. The symptoms of trauma remain. The dissociation remains. The threat might be gone, but the terrors and rage of trauma remain – perhaps for a lifetime, if unresolved.

Many people's legacy from traumatic events is an ongoing mass of unresolved emotions around the trauma. We can remain stuck. The dissociation remains the coping strategy. Ultimately, other, more appropriate strategies are required to replace the fallback position of dissociation. And, importantly, there is the need to move out of this dissociated stuckness. Levine writes that: "The way out of immobility is to experience it gradually, in relative safety, through the felt sense."

Let's not underestimate people's resilience and ingenuity. For example, when they are trapped and locked in an abusive relationship, or a personal fight for survival, or want to protect their children, they develop remarkable coping strategies, however tentative they might seem at the time. We can think of it in terms of survival, planning and escape.

Survival and coping mode: people have a great capacity to learn to adapt and respond, sometimes in unspeakably tough conditions.

Planning mode: developing plans and strategies to cope further. Beginning to consider strategies and tactics to escape an awful situation.

Escape mode: escaping the situation. This might mean giving up many things in exchange for freedom – perhaps a refuge instead of a home. And the abused individual might make several attempts at leaving before finally going through the door to freedom. Even then, they can be drawn back in. To an outsider, it might seem a conundrum – "*Why doesn't she just leave?*" But inside the relationship, it is often so difficult for the abusee to break free.

Ultimately, people will do whatever they need to do to survive and then to cope. And, crucially, do not to let the damage define you.

If you have been in a horrific situation or relationship, then remember this. However you cope and survive is your business, your creativity and yours alone. Many survivors develop ingenious and resilient coping mechanisms. There's no route map or satnav for finding your way out of these positions.

Each journey is individual; each journey is different. Connect your feet with the ground, take a few deep breaths and start walking. And keep walking.

Chapter 24

Get in touch with your core

We need to move the body as much as we move the mind.

I invite you to reflect on this question for a moment or two. Where is your core?

We have been exploring the brain, the heart and the gut. But where is your core?

Because we 'think', many people may consider and experience the core to be somewhere in the brain, between the ears. After all, that correlates with our eyes, and we see the world at head height through our eyes. We see, hear, smell, taste here, at head level. Yet we can feel anywhere in our body. Goosebumps can pop up all over the place. We sense things in our body.

For others, who are passionate and emotionally driven, perhaps they consider their core is their heart. Their feelings are very much to the fore as they go through life. They wear their hearts on their sleeves.

And we have also explored the gut and the gut 'brain'. We have recognised the value and power of gut instinct. Learning to trust our instinct, learning to trust our gut. We have explored the three brains approach – brain, heart and gut. But is there more? Where is the core?

A quick internet search using the words 'body core' will take you to an array of muscle-building, body-building websites. Add the word yoga, and you will discover an array of stretches, such as plank and bridge. Yoga is most definitely a route into the core.

Further research might take you to the psoas muscle, a remarkable muscle that is crucial to movement. It connects the upper body to the lower body, the inside to the outside and the back to the front. It extends from the spine over the pelvis to the femur in the leg. It works by flexing the hip joint, and it raises the upper leg to the body. Psoas muscles connect the spine to the legs. They are the deepest muscles in the core of the body.

Christiane Northrup contends that the psoas muscle "may be the most important muscle in your body". We are using it so often – to get up in the morning, walking, dancing, biking, bending. From sitting on a chair to exercising in yoga, it plays a role. And pretty important for sex too. It is a crucial 'enabler' muscle.

It has the potential to affect so many of our functions. We have already explored how we can hold tension in our chests that might restrict our ability to breathe and to communicate. Northrup writes that the psoas muscles are vital not just for our structural wellbeing but also for our psychological health due to their connection with the breath. What's more, when you are under stress, the psoas muscle can contract. Imagine what might happen in the trauma-induced fight, flight or freeze scenario.

Earlier in this book, I wrote about my traumatic experiences. Many years later, I was on the physiotherapist's table, having treatment for a sore back and lack of flexibility in my left hip. After I told the physiotherapist about my childhood experiences and my lack of flexibility, she asked me to lay flat on my back on the right-hand edge of the table and lower my right leg to the floor. I did this reasonably straightforwardly. She then asked me to repeat this exercise on the left side, using my left leg. As my leg lowered to the floor, my back arched upwards involuntarily. She told me to relax. I felt anxious, I didn't feel safe, as if I might fall. Gradually I repeated the exercise and, steadily, learnt to lower my leg in a more relaxed way.

I think that my muscles were still protecting me from an event that had happened decades earlier.

Liz Koch, an expert on the psoas muscle, contends that it has an important role in the fight, flight and freeze response to threat. She writes that it is perhaps this muscle that

"... provides the fear response its power to literally stop a person in his or her tracks. Considered an involuntary muscle, the psoas cannot therefore consciously be controlled. However, the psoas is a primal messenger of core integrity, survival, and informs a person when he or she is safe or in danger."

I only have a rudimentary understanding of the way the body works, but the words of Northrup and Koch, coupled with my own experiences simply seem to make sense – another couple of pieces of the jigsaw in my journey. And Northrup also writes that a psoas muscle imbalance can have a broad range of effects upon us – discrepancy in leg lengths; knee and lower back pain; postural problems; difficulty with bowel movements; menstrual cramps; shallow chest breathing and exhaustion.

The whole body is engaged when readying ourselves for the fight/flight/freeze response. That helps us if we run or fight, but what happens if we freeze, as can be experienced during a traumatic episode? And what happens if it is repeated? Koch contends that when the fear response is triggered repeatedly, the body can be left with perpetual tension. As we have explored earlier, we literally armour ourselves and internally dissociate. The consequence of this survival response, says Koch, is that "a deep sense of self is lost".

Hold a muscle tight and you will become tired quite quickly. Now consider the impact for the body if the psoas – one of the most important muscles in the body – is in a state of perpetual tension. Think about the energy that is used to hold that tension. It is exhausting. And how can the nervous system cope with this?

And this leaves me thinking about the breath. We have explored earlier in this book about the importance of breathing, but might the psoas muscles literally underlie the effects of shallow breath during times of stress? Pausing to breathe deeply and grounding ourselves is so helpful, but is there another layer to peel back? Do we need to release and energise the psoas muscles? And will this be liberating and allow us to move towards a healthier life?

As we explore the body in this way, we can see how much this might be a physiological issue as much as it is a psychological issue – perhaps even more so. This opens up new perspectives. If your psoas muscles aren't functioning and flowing freely, there may be significant impact elsewhere in you – both physically and psychologically. And if you have had a traumatic experience which triggered the fight/flight/freeze response, then your psoas might be carrying the tension within you. And think about that for a moment. Every step you take, every time you bend, stretch or make love – you could be carrying such additional, internalised 'invisible' tension.

Through listening to clients in the coaching room, I have often noticed their sheer levels of tension – and holding such tensions sucks in huge amounts of energy and interrupts the natural flow of the body.

We can consider our core from multiple, deeply interconnected places – whether the brain, the heart, the gut or the core muscles. Taking this perspective suggests that, as well as talking therapies, we can be engaging in physical therapies too. We need to get moving physically. We move the body as much as we move the mind.

Chapter 25

Boundaries: where I meet you and you meet me

You can change and I can change when we make contact at our boundary point.

There are some people who finish work, go home and leave their work behind. They won't do any further work until they go back the next day or the following week.

Then there are those who take work home, but only start work after dinner or when the children have gone to bed. They might open up their laptops for most of the evening. Others might put a time frame around this. One head teacher of a secondary school advised his staff that he stopped at nine o'clock at night. His message was that he didn't expect them to be working later than him. On some occasions, there may be urgent work that needs to be done, but it can also become something very regular. Some people might just take reading home with them. Others keep their laptops by the side of their beds.

If you have a job where there are possibilities for additional tasks, what are your boundaries? As can be seen from the examples above, some people maintain strict boundaries, while others have boundaries that are much more porous or even seemingly non-existent. It may be tied to a heightened sense of responsibility. Or dissatisfaction of not doing a good enough job. And there is a question to be explored around boundaries – what is healthy, and what is unhealthy?

Your boundary here is your 'contact' point. Think of it in terms of three contact points:

- Your relationship with the task.
- Your relationship with other people – perhaps work colleagues or family at home.
- Your relationship with yourself – in the context of work and more broadly.

Here's an example of contact with a task. Perhaps you are a workaholic – or know someone who is. They work and work all day and through the evening – but it never seems quite enough. There is always something more they could have done – or achieved to a higher standard. They have powerful contact with their work but get little satisfaction – perhaps even dissatisfaction – from their outputs. Their relationship with themselves is a harsh one. The quality of the contact with themselves, through critical self-talk, is not healthy. It's never quite enough. It's never satisfying. So they drive themselves on to work harder, yet still not able to achieve satisfaction. It would help these people not only to address the amount of work they do, but also their relationship with work and the erroneous perceived quality they have of work. Some people just work harder and harder to avoid the anxieties of possible failure. Such behaviours in adult life will often have started from difficulties during childhood – perhaps where the sense of not being good enough all began.

You might wish to consider what your boundaries are like. Work is just one example of this. And notice how the examples above derive from earlier experiences. Our patterns of work may replicate those of our parents – or perhaps a rebellion against those. Or expectations put upon us by our parents and our school environment.

You can also think about boundaries and contact points in many other areas – perhaps in relationships or the ability to say 'no'. Notice how you are with other people. Is yours an open house or a private place? We encounter each other at our contact point – the boundary edge between two people.

People who have experienced traumatic incidents may find their boundaries are much less certain. Perhaps boundaries are more open and porous. Perhaps they feel they're being taken advantage of but can't quite put their finger on it. Or perhaps they're the one staying late in the office most days of the week.

We can also think of the physical contact point that exists with others too. As we explored earlier, your skin is your contact point between you and your environment – whether objects or people. James Kepner describes the following example of human contact through touch. Imagine someone touches you on the shoulder while your muscles are tense. And then repeat the exercise when your muscles are relaxed. The 'contact' in the first instance is shallow; in the second it is different, deeper. You are more open for meaningful touch, for meaningful contact with another person.

How are your muscles on a general day-to-day basis? This softer boundary leads you to be more receptive to the other person's touch – and more vulnerable. In a loving relationship, this is healthy and offers opportunities for growth through contact, but the permeability might also act as a physical intrusion, perhaps regenerating former traumatic experiences. In which case, your fight, flight or freeze responses might be triggered. A muscle's purpose is to tense or relax. And we do need muscular tension – otherwise we couldn't get up and walk about.

What is the boundary that works for you? Boundaries are developed and shaped by each individual – by you.

Think about your boundaries:

- I don't let anyone get really close to me. *Or* I have many close friends.
- I only trust a few people. *Or* I trust many different people.
- People walk all over me. *Or* Nobody walks over me.
- I feel a bit like a doormat. *Or* People are welcome to my home, but the boundaries are clear.
- I let people get away with murder. *Or* I do not let people take advantage of me.

It will help to reflect upon the psychological and physical boundaries and the relationship between them.

Firstly, consider the following question:

Are your boundaries reactive or responsive?

- Reactive, as if you are on autopilot? "I can't say no."
- Responsive, when and where you are choosing your boundaries. "I am comfortable saying 'no' without giving a reason."

In the reactive position, the trauma survivor might be just repeating patterns of the traumatised event(s) – perhaps inappropriately close with people or too isolated.

Thinking about these will help to build your self-awareness. And observe if, for example, your ability to say 'no' differs from one situation to another. I have noticed, for example, that many people find it easier to say 'no' in the following situations:

- Professionally rather than personally.
- Saying no on behalf of others rather than themselves.

If this applies to you, then you have the capacity to say 'no' in certain contexts. Perhaps your journey is to strengthen this capacity across more areas of your life – personally as well as professionally; on behalf of yourself and not just others.

In the responsive position, the respondent comes from a position of choice. If it is you, then you have put in place a boundary. You have learnt to say 'no' to people. And remember two of the golden threads that run through this book:

- Awareness is so important.
- You always have the key in your pocket.

Activity

Reflect upon a personal boundary issue.

- Identify the boundary topic.
- Are you coming from a reactive or responsive position?
- What do you notice?

• Identify the boundary topic.
• Are you coming from a reactive or responsive position?
• What do you notice?

Now I invite you to imagine two positions, the reactive and the responsive.

• When coming from a reactive position, how do you feel?
• Now imagine you are coming from a responsive position; how do you feel?

And finally, ask yourself the following:

• Given a fresh start, how might you choose to respond differently?

Chapter 26

Karen's story: from nursing and waiting to coaching and changing

If you work with a therapist or a coach, you might experience them as someone who is calm, supportive, empathic and replete in emotional intelligence.

That's often the case. Yet they might have been on a long personal journey to arrive at this place. It's not uncommon for coaches and therapists to start their journeys on the other side of the table – as clients rather than as experts.

Responsible and effective coaches will have done a lot of work on their own 'stuff', to increase their self-awareness and the value they can add to their clients.

Karen is one of these. I first met Karen in the setting of the Institute of Continuing Education, part of the University of Cambridge. I was course director of their coaching programmes, and Karen wanted to undertake her coach training journey. [I am the tutor she describes in her story.]

We talked together, and I experienced her as someone with great sensitivity, empathy and warmth. Fortunately, she chose to train as a coach and the rest, as the saying goes, is history. Since establishing her professional coaching practice, she has co-authored a coaching book with two other former students.

She kindly chose to share her story, and I hope you find it to be as engaging, courageously honest and as ultimately inspiring as I do.

Here is Karen's story.

From nursing and waiting to coaching and changing

Karen shares her journey through different traumatic experiences in a conversation with Keith.

After working for 30 years as a registered nurse, the hospital I worked in closed. The handling of this event in 2012 by the Health Trust made the process very painful. We had a meeting to say it would close, together with the planned date, a few months away. Even though we knew it was coming, everyone felt shell-shocked.

Two days later, a subsequent emergency meeting informed us that the hospital would shut immediately after Easter, and the staff would be dispersed to other hospitals. We were left to make sense of this over the long weekend while the Trust's leaders took their Easter break.

There was no one to talk to and no support. The union appeared to be siding with the Trust and not the nurses.

It did not make sense; the hospital provided a much-needed service; where would these patients go? The hospital provided a vital step-up and step-down service. Step-up for patients unable to cope in the home environment, but not suitable to be admitted into the acute setting. Step-down meant they were ready to leave the acute setting but not fit for home. It was a much-needed and valued unit. The Trust informed us that we still had our jobs but would need to apply for other positions and be interviewed; everything seemed contradictory.

Having devoted my whole working life to nursing, I know that nurses are used to constant change. Every shift is different; there is always a variety of patients with varying illness, collective colleagues working different shift patterns, so teams are different every day. There is a continuous flow of change, adapting and learning.

But even with this flexibility around working, the effect on patients and staff alike from this imposed change was devastating.

So after 30 years working as a nurse in a hospital, you were told it would close. The leaders were away; there was no one to talk to, and a lack of support from the union. You still had a job, but you would have to apply for a new position. And working in a caring profession, no one seemed to be concerned for you. You described it as "devastating" and that you and your colleagues felt "shell-shocked". What was life like during those first few weeks, and how did you cope?

I felt incredibly alone, and it seemed my whole world was ripped away from me. I was wide-eyed in front of car lights, frozen, bewildered, frightened and unable to comprehend.

I was a nurse first and foremost; I now know this is what had held me together for years.

I became more and more overwhelmed. To others, my behaviour changed (my mum even thought I was on "something"). It was as if I just sped up. I developed physical, unexplained pain, especially in my legs.

Crying was a big part of me at that time. If I could be in nature, I felt more able to cope, but as soon as I was back in 'reality', I struggled. I was unable to function. I withdrew. There is little I can remember other than the emotion I felt.

What was the worst part of those weeks?

- No one able to understand – that's not to say they didn't try.
- I was unable to make sense of it – the facility was so important and much needed.
- Tears upon tears – how can this be happening?
- Lonely – and a loss of purpose. I felt disregarded and disrespected. (Most of my values were being trodden on.)

- Grief – I loved my job, loved my patients, loved leading teams, loved learning, loved mentoring. Work had been like a family.
- Not being able to make a difference anymore.
- Being sent to another hospital that was to close shortly too. It felt like "let's do it again to her". Where would I eventually end up?

Karen, you say that nursing had "held me together for years". Was there other trauma that you had previously experienced?

Nursing was a constant for me. I felt in control and respected. People noticed I did a good job and that I was reliable for my patients, students and colleagues. When I felt needed, then I felt that I mattered.

My childhood had been difficult. My dad was an alcoholic, and when drink became his focus, the dad I worshipped no longer noticed me anymore. As my dad's drinking progressed, he started having accidents, bleeds and other problems – so I was always with him in the hospital setting – I spent many hours waiting, which I later realised would have a significant impact upon me.

I was a sad child who didn't feel safe at home or school; I didn't realise that until many years later when I trained to become a professional life coach.

My nursing took me away from my home environment. I found being kind and helpful to the vulnerable meant I got noticed. I felt their vulnerability. Caring for them helped me to feel fulfilled and to have my sense of purpose. I felt at ease and enjoyed the hospital environment.

Was there any other trauma? What patterns did you notice?

Along with the imposed traumas throughout my childhood, I also have had imposed trauma in my married life. Stephen, my husband, has a love for motorbikes and speed, but as he has got older and with injuries, he has become more susceptible to accidents. Many of these accidents have been major trauma, which required extensive metalwork repair for his many broken bones.

I was aware I seemed to be always visiting hospitals, waiting for Stephen to get better. I later became aware of how busy I had been. The image is trying to keep lids on all my boxes; periodically, I would be given the biggest box with the top right off, belonging once to my dad and now to my husband. Many a person had said to me: "I don't know how you do all you do." I now listen to the observations of others. I began to take a step back and revaluate.

What I noticed was that I was found myself in the same trauma, but just with a different person. [My coaching would later help me cope.]

What about the pain you described in your legs?

The physical pain came on as soon as I moved to a different hospital. It was a small cottage hospital with staff that didn't care, who just sat around instead of getting on with the work. I sped up to compensate when I was already nearly on my knees. The pain was my body trying to make me stop; this is when I saw the GP as I knew I couldn't go on.

You say that in the early weeks you were "frozen, bewildered, frightened". If we think of it in terms of fight, flight or freeze, I'm hearing "frozen", but not fight or flight. Was this the case?

I was in flight until the death of a family member, and then I froze, I collapsed, I withdrew into my head, I struggled to function, to do normal things. The only one thing that remained constant was going to look after the old family pony. I would stay with him as long as I could, but as soon as I drove away, I would start to cry again.

You say that you couldn't go on. What happened?

It was like the last straw. My mind and body were stopping me from functioning. I believe because I couldn't make sense of the experience, I became so overwhelmed that I shut down. My mind made me stop by giving me physical pain, and I couldn't function as the pain overwhelmed me. I had immense tiredness too. I remember I kept thinking, "I can't do this."

All my nursing principles were being challenged. There was also another very difficult situation to handle, which involved a narcissistic person. Without going into detail, the lack of empathy for another human being was unbelievable. I have an understanding of the fear of being present with such a person.

Were you able to keep working?

I stopped working from July. I never went back to nursing but remained employed by the Trust until the autumn when I was diagnosed with bilateral breast cancer.

[I am involved in my husband's business. I worked there since 2003, became a partner in 2016, and on the sudden death of our young partner in 2017, I stepped up to take on more roles.]

What happened then? And how did you start to move forwards?

Between July and autumn, I did very little, still processing what had happened. I walked in nature with my daughter's dog, and I noticed everything in great detail. I was doing my best to heal.

When I got my diagnosis with cancer, this started the nurturing stage. I just let the doctors and nurses look after me. I felt that I mattered. I didn't research anything, just trusted the staff and went along with whatever they decided was the best plan of action.

Death didn't frighten me. If it was my time, I was okay with that.

I was offered coaching at the end of the treatment, and I knew I needed to grasp this opportunity. It was like a shining light. I used this time to make sense of the experience I had at the end of my nursing. There were lots of tears, but I was moving forward. Towards the end of the sessions, I realised I could become a coach, and I could support people without being a nurse. I had a vision for my new sense of purpose.

I was also becoming aware of how other people were getting their work done; at a slower pace, and that was okay. I had been at near burnout for years. It felt like I was rushing at everything, but it was my mind rather than my body that heightened sense of data. People have always said I have a calming influence; I didn't feel it even though I showed it. Now, most of the time, I feel calm.

With my new sense of purpose, I attended an open day which introduced me to a coach training programme. I was still raw and scared. I had struggled academically at school, but my determination to regain my sense of purpose meant I would push forward.

So, to sum up so far, Karen, you had an alcoholic father who "no longer noticed me anymore"; a husband who had multiple motorcycle accidents; a hospital that took you away from your home environment and became your purpose – but which was then abruptly and brutally closed; a new hospital where the staff didn't care; and then the diagnosis of breast cancer. You were the common denominator in this, and separately you told me that: "I always have a sense I am waiting to be allowed to do anything out of the house." Can you tell me more about that, about you – where the internalised need for permission came from and the impact it had on you?

As a child, I would ask my dad permission to do something with friends and then later I would be told off, sometimes harshly, for going and doing it; I didn't know where I stood.

We were always waiting for dad to come home so we could have dinner. Standing at the window waiting. (I now understand, from writing this, why I feel I am waiting now, my husband is always running late, I stand at the window and wait; the accidents, waiting for him to get better and life to return to normal.) For me, the act of waiting brings on sadness and loneliness.

As I have grown over the last eight years, I am less tolerant of waiting and less likely to do it. Nowadays, I will move forward by taking the lead, so I am not waiting anymore.

Can you explain why and how the following were important and beneficial for you:

Time spent with your horse and your daughter's dog.

Being with animals means that the demands made of me are removed, so I can focus on what is, without interruption. My view is undisturbed. I am sensitive to the data around me. Being in nature, with animals, is soothing, warming and enjoyable.

Your running.

Freedom, challenge, wellbeing, solitude, outside in the light, and part of nature.

The benefit of simply allowing yourself to be taken care of by the medical staff.

I had been seen, I was worthy of kindness, nothing was expected of me, I could just be still. I have always given to people what I have wanted myself; I realise that now. I don't need to be in the limelight; I just need to be noticed when I am present.

I remember you [Keith] saying to me there is a little girl inside you trying to get out. That little girl has been able to grow into an adult over the last few years and is learning how to just be.

Acceptance is easier now; coaching study has shown me to accept what *was* and *is*. Letting go of what I can't control and concentrating on what I can. It has given me the ability to continue in my development to bring about change for me. The wisdom of understanding the story, why I responded the way I did, how it was for anyone else in any situation.

How did coaching help you when you were ill? What impact did it have for you?

Coaching's impact was immense, and it enabled me to start making sense of my overwhelming reaction to my work experience. The homework I had gave me focus and I learnt a lot about myself. I grew stronger and began to see a future, a place for me to be supporting others. Again, I felt that I mattered, and it's okay to have feelings and express them.

I realised what my values were, and that all of them had been trodden on by my experiences at the end of my nursing career. That was the reason the experience was so overwhelming. Now I can see when it is happening and have the choice to remove myself from the situation. I sense it very quickly in my body and understand what those feelings are about – a very precious insight.

It seems that helping others is integral with you. What made you decide to become a coach, and how has it helped you?

To coach is to support. Feeling the experience of being coached inspired me to be able to learn something new. It was gentle, unrushed and positively productive.

I knew I couldn't return to nursing because I put everything into it without considering myself. It is hard work mentally and physically, and I no longer had that stamina.

Through my study, I have gotten to know myself better. I consider myself in every equation and give myself choice. Even if I don't choose the one that would be best for me, I have the awareness of what I am doing. I have developed the somatic approach, where every aspect of a person is reunited and attuned. The rushing world of today has caused people to lose sight of themselves. I am hopeful that on the other side of this virus, we will take forward our lessons to make the world a better place for every living creature, we will nurture and care for life.

There has been such a rise in coaching in the last few years. I originally thought that it was to clear the hatred, but now I believe it is here to heal, change and make connections of love and kindness.

Can you please tell me some more about the somatic approach? You mention "reunited" and "attuned".

Starting with meditation provides space to reconnect with my body and to experience what my body is sharing.

The ability to reconnect with my body, to listen and act to provide self-care. This learning and its importance I share with my clients. It brings me the gift of being present with myself. It enables clients to be present to their selves.

Through re-uniting, one reconnects to one's self emotionally, physically and spiritually. Attunement allows one to be in harmony and aligned.

When you look back on your traumatic journey, what have been the critical factors that have allowed you to overcome the trauma and to enable you to become the person you are today? What have you done and how have you been?

- The constant presence of nature.
- My family just let me be; they had never seen me broken and probably didn't know what to do.
- Having cancer gave me the nurturing and time to heal my trauma – the start of my recovery.
- Being coached – to process my trauma, make sense of it and the discovery of a way forward to develop a new sense of purpose. A challenge, to improve me in ways I did not feel I was capable of – study and assignments.
- Coaching course – more understanding of my trauma and me as a person. Keith, my tutor, sensing my vulnerability, who gently challenged me. The people I shared the study with – and I still connect with many of them. The knowledge that it's okay to express how I feel.

- I am good enough.
- To become responsive rather than reactive.
- The ability to sit in ambiguity.
- I notice and understand the reactions of others with more clarity. I have learnt not to take other people's outbursts personally because it is about them, not me.
- My confidence has increased, I can manage any challenge, and I have acknowledged all I have achieved in my life.
- I feel at one when connecting with like-minded people, especially with interest in the somatic approach and trauma coaching. I attend webinars with hundreds of people, listening, learning and experiencing the calmness of coaches.
- I feel happy and content now, I sense in my body if things are not right for me, and I do my best to make changes. As in anyone's life, sometimes it is a long process due to the complexity of the situation. I was starting to come out of my trauma through my study, so felt particularly vulnerable and over-challenged at times, but I would not have done it any differently. My learning has been immense, welcomed and thankful. I am feeling strong, capable and unstoppable in achieving my dreams.
- I love to witness others developing, growing awareness and finding their new way of being; it brings so much happiness to me and them alike.

How important has been your growing self-awareness?

Growing self-awareness has been the golden nugget, the key to becoming the new me. It gives a wealth of knowledge of what makes me tick, how to develop that understanding for more significant learning, observing myself and my interactions with others; I now have a deep curiosity. Self-awareness is an enabler to grow as a unique individual for empowered and positive outcomes and to continue that self-awareness with regular reflection.

Can you give an example of how your raised awareness has enabled you to change one of your behaviours in a way that has worked for you?

My awareness to always say 'yes' to everything asked of me without considering if it is right for me has changed. I pause and think before I answer the request if I sense it is not right for me; I am now comfortable in saying 'no'. It took me a long time to develop this, but it is so good to have that choice.

Another awareness is that it is okay for me to sit and rest, to be in the moment. Before, I would not rest, I always had to be seen to be doing.

Confidence in my ability to learn and feel fulfilled in new learnings. I can achieve, and I am up for the challenge.

What advice would you give to someone who is struggling from the memories of a traumatic experience in their life?

- Find the right support.
- Be loving and kind to yourself and how you feel. Your experience of a traumatic event is a normal response to something painful and life-changing. It is hard to process quickly.
- What will make you feel nurtured? Connect for your wellbeing.
- Give yourself time to rest, sleep and exercise.
- Notice nature, study what you are seeing, look at the beauty around you.
- The use of an emotional diary can help with the healing process.
- Focus on what sensations you feel inside yourself, along with meditation techniques to help clear your mind and release built-up energy from the trauma.
- What is the support you need? Is it friends, family or a trauma specialist?

- If you feel overwhelmed by the experience, then reach out to a trauma specialist therapist or coach. Have a conversation with several to find the one that you feel is a safe connection.
- In time, start to take back control of the things you can control; this is a big part of moving forward.
- Understand your values – and living by them will give you inner peace and guidance when something does sit well for you.

Finally, Karen, could you summarise your journey from who you were as a nurse to how you are now as a life coach in a single sentence?

My eyes are wide open to the possibilities on offer in life, and I am intrigued to see what is there for me; I am no longer hiding behind the image of a nurse and what that represents; I now support others in their challenge to change.

PART 4

Relief through release: why listening is so important

This is a short but important section in this book – it's fundamental to the value of listening to understand. From the position of the person who has been through a very difficult time, being listened to – and really heard – is so important. It is core to the relationship between therapist and client.

There is so much to be gained from a listening-based conversation. When we really listen to someone, when we give them our full attention, our full presence, then we are giving the other person a wonderful gift. It is so crucial to enable people who have experienced difficult times to process their experiences and to feel lighter on their journeys forward.

This chapter explores what can go wrong – when the conversation is less about listening to the other, and more about giving advice and seeking to solve the other person's problems. The following chapter considers the benefits of just listening to the other person.

If you have experienced trauma and find that others don't really understand you and your situation, then you might wish to share these chapters with them.

It boils down to three words: relief through release.

Good listening!

CHAPTER 27

Being listened to or being given advice? What you don't want

The problem with someone who knows best for you is that, very probably, they don't.

I believe there is a very curious, and very true, paradox in life. And it's this. It's seemingly so much easier to solve other people's problems than it is your own. I don't know if you've noticed this?

We seem to be a nation – if not a whole world – of problem-solvers. By and large, we can quickly have lots of ideas to solve others' problems for them. It seems to be so easy. Somehow, our own problems seem much more intractable.

When I train people to become coaches, I encourage them not to set out to solve the other's problem or to seek to 'fix' them. This seems counter-intuitive. After all, it is a natural human trait to want to help others, so the intent is good. And, generally, people do like to tell, advise, offer support, guide, direct, solve… you name it, we do it. We don't like to see others in a state of discomfort. Yet this advice brings with it challenges, which might include the following. It can:

- Imply that the person is not capable of solving the 'issue'.
- Disempower.
- Patronise.
- Infantilise.
- Minimise.

Too often, it just repeats previous messages the person might have heard. And often the advice comes from the other's perspective. To be blunt, it reflects the old saying that mummy – or daddy – knows best.

With the best will in the world, if we are trying to solve the other's problem, too often we are doing so from our perspective. Not their perspective. Maybe to exert some sort of control over the situation. Maybe to steer ourselves away from our own discomfort. We don't like to see others in a place of discomfort, and consequently we feel uncomfortable ourselves. Therefore, if we can 'fix' their problem, we feel more comfortable in ourselves – we ease our own sense of discomfort.

Being given advice – or told what to do

How often have you heard the following? Below is a table of statements that you might be familiar with – that you might have heard. I have categorised them:

- Handling emotions.
- Giving advice.
- Attempting to take over.

In the right-hand column, you can read how these statements might be interpreted. You may have your own responses too!

On handling emotions

What the person giving advice might say	How it might be heard by the receiver
Man up.	I am weak.
Pull yourself together.	I didn't know I was falling apart. I must have fallen apart.
It can't be that bad.	Maybe I'm making a mountain out of a molehill.

Cheer up.	I didn't know I was miserable.
Be strong.	I'm obviously not strong.
Remember: stiff upper lip.	How do I do that?

Giving advice

What the 'adviser' says	How it might be heard
You need to.	If you say so. Do I need to?
Try this.	I tried that already. It didn't work then. Do I have to try it again?
If you do this, then.	Not sure about that, really.
Why don't you…?	Why should I?
You'll get over it.	How do you know? Will I?
You should…	Here we go again, someone telling me what I 'should' do.

Attempting to take over

What the 'adviser' says	How it might be heard
If I was you, I would…	That's what my father used to say… (And I never liked what he said anyway.)
I know exactly how you feel.	Do you? How do you know how I feel?
The same thing happened to me.	Did it? You always turn the conversation back onto you.

Let me say one thing.	Here we go again. Heard it all before.
The same thing happened to a friend of mine, and she is perfectly okay.	For heaven's sake, leave me alone.

As you read through the statements in the left-hand column, all sorts of responses might be triggered in the right column.

What makes this clumsy and intrusive advice worse is that the person receiving 'advice' may well be coming from a position of vulnerability. They will have heard such phrases before. Sometimes even from the perpetrator of the trauma. So, the speaker's advice often leads to feelings such as inferiority, incapability, inability… and so on. Advice often backfires.

And it can get worse. Sometimes the adviser becomes frustrated or even takes offence because the recipient hasn't responded in the way they expected!

The person dealing with the aftermath of traumatic experiences will benefit from something different.

To be listened to, to be heard and to be understood.

We will explore this theme in the following chapter.

CHAPTER 28

When what you really want is just to be heard and understood

Never forget that really being listened to is a fundamental human need.

Never underestimate the value of simply being listened to and, to some degree, understood. There's an old saying:

A problem shared is a problem halved.

Notice the simplicity of those words – sharing the problem. (Not fixing them.)

Being listened to, really feeling that you have been heard, is so important. Everyone has a story to tell, so we can at least listen to it. Certainly, those with traumatic experiences and memories have stories to tell.

Having the space to be able to talk about the story is so important. In therapy, clients will visit and re-visit their stories. (The therapist creates an environment for the client to do so safely.) Talking out loud brings things from the subconscious to the conscious. New perspectives can be achieved.

There is a wonderful relief from release – being able to talk things through. Without interruptions, without being given advice, without someone seeking to fix you, without being told what to do, without feeling belittled, without being judged. Back in 1961, Carl Rogers proposed that the "major barrier to mutual interpersonal communication is our very natural tendency to judge, to evaluate, to approve or disapprove, the statement of the other person."

Rogers was a therapist. Most of us aren't therapists. Yet we can listen.

- Offloading in this way is cathartic.
- Talking out loud, comfortably, is therapeutic, without being therapy.
- Never underestimate just how powerful deep listening can be.

There's another wonderful saying:

Getting it off your chest.

That simple pleasure of being allowed to get things off your chest – feeling comfortable to talk freely with an empathic listener.

And, of course, getting things off your chest implies things are on your chest. Just imagine that something is on your chest. Its weight compresses your breathing. Your supply of oxygen is restricted. It feels tight. Many people hold tension in and around their chest. Sharing a problem allows you to release this weight off your chest.

Having heard clients share their challenges over many years, I have come to appreciate that the simple act of listening – and really hearing someone – is, simply, priceless. I don't think it's possible to put a value on it. It's a wonderful gift to the other person.

Have you ever paused to consider the benefits for the speaker when they are really listened to?

When clients have shared their traumatic experiences, they can experience the following:

What happens for the speaker when they have been really listened to	The impact this can have for the speaker
They have often opened up in a way that they have never done before with anyone else.	Wow! Surprise! Where did all that come from? That felt a bit risky, and I'm self-conscious because I cried a few times. Hope I didn't seem stupid.
They sense that they have really been heard for the first time.	That was good. I didn't get interrupted. He just listened to me and asked me a few questions. I haven't talked so much in ages. The time flew by.
They might have spoken about it before with well-meaning friends or relatives, but who had started giving advice.	It was good not to be told what to do and what not to do. That made a change. Such a relief.
They feel understood or partially understood.	At last! Somebody seems to understand me and what I've been going through.
They feel validated. Often for the first time in their life.	I didn't get judged or criticised. Being understood has validated my experiences and my feelings.
They feel less isolated.	It isn't just me! I really thought this was only happening to me.
They realise they are not going mad. "I thought it was me going crazy."	I'm not mad. For years I wondered if I was going mad. Now I realise it's not me.

The overall impact of this type of discussion – of opening up for the first time – can be an immense release through relief.

The simple activity of speaking and being listened to is a wonderful process of unburdening. Earlier we discussed the truth behind some very traditional phrases. Here's another:

A weight off your shoulders.

People can carry their traumatic – and other – experiences – as a real weight. Perhaps they bear a huge sense of responsibility:

- For the decisions they made.
- Or that they couldn't help another person more.
- Or that they made "mistakes".
- Or that it was their fault.

These can easily become millstones such as guilt and/or shame. Carrying the weight of secrets. Over a period of weeks, months, years or decades, these might have sat with them on their shoulders. It might take many conversations to process these feelings and lighten the burden. Being listened to, empathically, and without judgement, is crucial on the journey.

John Gray, in *Men are from Mars, women are from Venus* proposes the two most common mistakes that people make in relationships.

- For men to women, he described how men try to change women's feelings when they are upset by making suggestions. He proposed this would "invalidate her feelings".
- And women, he argued, would try to change men's behaviours by offering "unsolicited advice or criticism".

Those wise words were written nearly 30 years ago – they remain rich to this day.

Let's just listen. Listen to really hear. Listen to understand.

Activity

Listening and being listened to

Think about who you might be able to talk to about your experiences. This may be a therapist. Yet a trusted friend or loved one can also be a great support.

- Who could you talk to?
- What makes this person suitable?
- Agree a 'behaviour' contract before you start. Let them know what you want.

For those listening to someone talk about their trauma:

- How can you show up as a listener?
- How can you best create the space for the talker?
- Agree a 'behaviour' contract before you start.

CHAPTER 29

Rob's story: from near-death to rebirth to physical and creative growth

I have known Rob pretty well nearly all his life – he is my nephew. A few years ago, when he was aged 34, disaster struck. Not only did he suffer very badly from a burst appendix, but his marriage also came to an end.

Here, we will read Rob's account of his journey through his illness and then recovery – from recuperation to renewal to regeneration.

I write elsewhere in this book of my belief that many – if not most – people experience traumatic episode(s) through their lives. Indeed, Rob is not the only close relative I could have invited to share their stories.

Here's what happened…

From near-death to rebirth to physical and creative growth

Please give me an overview of the traumatic event – what happened.

On Monday 31 July 2017, I started to feel really sick. By the Thursday of that week, I was in so much pain that I could not walk and felt like I had no option but to call for an ambulance.

The doctor later told me that had I waited a further hour to do this, then I would have died.

My appendix had burst, leaking poison into my body and giving me sepsis. The surgeon told me that the state of my stomach had been so bad that the extent of the chemical cleaning they'd had to do in surgery resulted in internal chemical burns to 50% of my body.

I was unable to walk, go to the toilet or shower unassisted and was very sick.

After leaving hospital, my marriage started to break down very quickly, and after three weeks, I had to leave the family home. Consequently, I then had to deal with the trauma of what had happened to me, cope with recovering from nearly dying alongside the trauma of my marriage break-up and divorce.

What was life like during those first few weeks, and how did you cope?

Everything had completely changed. Truthfully, I am not sure how I coped – other than to say that some kind of inbuilt survival mechanism kicked in that I cannot really hope to communicate to others who haven't been in that position.

I was not able to walk when I left hospital, so I had to be pushed out in a wheelchair. I passed out in the car on the drive home; I vividly remember the noise of the car, the other cars, the road, the weather and the over-stimulation of my senses which had been dulled by a week in a hospital bed. The seatbelt was agony to put on over my chest. It took 45 minutes to get me from the car into the house, as I could not walk and was so weak. I remember it was raining biblically – like something out of a movie.

I was so glad initially to be back at home in my own space and not in hospital, but it took time to adjust. I would wake up frequently, unable to sleep for long periods, and when I did wake up, I was always soaked in sweat. I could not move my arms or legs and didn't know where I was. It would take me about 15 minutes each time to understand that I was not in hospital or still dreaming. I would then have to be lifted out of the bed and helped to the toilet. The bedroom was upstairs, so each day it was a mission to climb up and down the stairs.

At first my dad physically lifted me, but gradually I was able to crawl up them and then ultimately climb up them myself, but it took a monumental effort.

The trouble was that my brain knew how to walk upstairs, but my body couldn't, so it became very frustrating. If I tried to do it too quickly, I could easily tire and get distressed – and not be able to go any further. It took a long time to relearn how to walk and to climb up stairs.

Ultimately, I found that playing my favourite music (in particular *Rage Against the Machine*) really helped with tasks like this.

I couldn't eat properly and could only handle a very small amount of mashed-up food that would take a very long time to swallow. I couldn't really focus on anything properly for long periods of time – so I ended up watching the same films over and over again.

I was heavily reliant on other people, and looking back at the whole scope of my recovery now that I am physically fit again, I view this period as though I was a baby – in the sense that I needed help in essentially all the ways a baby does.

To stick with the theme – this really did feel like a period of rebirth for me, too, as I was feeling like a different person to who I was before I got sick.

What was the worst part of those weeks?

I am not really comfortable discussing this publicly, but in the interest that this might be of use to someone else further down the line, I will, in broad strokes.

Aside from the obvious physical pain, the worst part of these weeks was the misunderstanding of my condition that certain people showed.

I guess to some people when someone comes out of hospital, they can view that person as now being 'better' – as they no longer need hospitalisation. I know from personal experience that this is absolutely not the case. Leaving hospital was really just the first step in a marathon towards full recovery.

But when, for example, your broken leg is not in plaster, or there is no visible wound, and your illness is internal and cannot be viewed by people, other than the state that you are in – I guess it's harder for people to sympathise or empathise with your pain, a pain they cannot visualise. Unfortunately, this was my experience.

To be clear, I was in a lot of physical pain for a very long time. (Illness, appendicitis, sepsis, keyhole surgery and internal chemical burns over the space of a few days.) The medical advice given to me by multiple professionals was to treat the pain – I therefore was on painkillers as much as I was allowed, as it was very much required.

However, certain people close to me said things such as, "You're not going to recover if you keep taking painkillers", and further words to that effect. Which, when you're desperately reliant on the painkillers to give you just a few minutes of feeling slightly more human before the pain kicks in again, are not words that are conducive to a healthy recovery environment.

Needless to say, tensions escalated, my condition stayed the same and actually worsened despite me trying every day to push myself further than I had done the previous day. Ultimately, I had to leave the family home as I was simply not able to recover there.

So where did you go, Rob, and how did you start that long journey to recovery?

The only place I was able to go after all this and in the state that I was in was back to my parents' house. After what I had experienced, this represented a 'safe place' to me, where I was finally able to feel that it was OK to focus solely on my recovery and getting better.

Starting on the journey of recovery consisted of a few things. With the benefit of hindsight and looking back, I now recognise that acceptance of what had happened to me was a key factor.

I am not sure how long it took to accept my circumstances, but when I ultimately did this, it aided me in my attempt to get fit and healthy. I walked, I read, I built Lego, I played my guitar, I wrote music, I found solace in familiar movies and old WWE [wrestling] pay per views – anything I could do to take my mind off the trauma of what had happened.

Physically I did whatever I felt like I could do in that day. This was mainly walking a few steps up and down the garden, but this would ultimately progress to walking around the block, to walking in the woods around the house. I was hindered in this effort as a couple of weeks after returning home, I was admitted back to hospital – with an abscess in an inoperable area, meaning I needed another five days in hospital.

I came out of there, though, with renewed purpose, probably thinking that the worst was over. Now that the infection was gone, I could get better.

Again, I kept moving as much as I could and gradually worked my way back to walking around again. I walked every single day without fail, keenly aware that I needed to get my stamina and strength back. Some days it was especially hard, and some days were different. It didn't matter if it was raining or bright sunshine – I still walked.

After about six weeks, this progressed to being able to walk in the swimming pool – which again I did without fail every day. After another few weeks, this progressed to very light swimming, which I continued to do as much as I could. This wasn't necessarily as easy as it sounds – throughout this time I was still on painkillers and still feeling very sick, although gradually over time this started to get better. However, I still consistently had pains in my chest for a very long time.

Rob, it's now two years since you fell ill. How are you now, and what other things are you doing to keep well?

I am now physically much stronger than I have ever been. In April 2018 (about nine months after surgery) when I finally felt able to, I started going to the gym, and since then I haven't stopped. The gym was very close by, so I was able to go almost every lunchtime; in general, at least five times a week.

Before getting sick, I had never been to a gym, and always felt intimidated by it. But when I was in hospital, I was acutely aware of my body (more so than ever before). I had a very strong desire that when I was able to, I would go to the gym and get myself fit.

There is a great Conor McGregor quote – *"movement is medicine"* – and that really resonated with me at the time.

I found the gym to be a place of solace, somewhere I could go anytime, and for the amount of time I was working out – that was the only focus in my brain. My entire being, body and mind, was purely focused on getting that activity done, getting those 10 reps in or whatever it might be. It was also a place to continually push myself and see results both in terms of my health and what I was able to do and see progress week after week. In that sense, it's very addictive. I felt then – and still do – that I now have an advantage at the gym, in the sense that I never need any motivation to go – and actually enjoy my time there.

There is nothing more motivating than remembering what it was like to not be able to walk, and to have been that sick – and to have been through what I have. From that point of view, a tough workout in the gym is a walk in the park.

I also started taking up yoga – my brother is a yoga teacher at the gym, so going to his classes was a no-brainer. Again, I found that doing an exercise I was unfamiliar with regularly became routine and then habit and was then ultimately massively beneficial to my

177

overall wellbeing. I also focused on food and eating healthily – I haven't had an alcoholic drink since I was sick. The thinking here is that I do not want to knowingly put anything into my body that I know has the potential to make me feel ill. Having been very sick in the past, I never want to go anywhere near that again if I can possibly avoid it.

What have been the key factors for you in your ongoing recovery? From that time when you literally had to get back on your feet?

I started going to counselling very early on – I think that helped exponentially. Looking back, perhaps that helped more with the emotional aspects (divorce etc.), whereas the gym helped more with the physical aspects (sepsis/surgery/recovery). But they overlapped a lot.

In the times between counselling sessions, I could feel stuff boiling up and would almost count down the days to the next appointment. Sometimes I came out feeling better, sometimes worse – but always moving forward. Mainly I think my counsellor helped me with the sense of guilt I felt at leaving, to not be so hard on myself and also that what had happened wasn't my fault.

Aside from that, after about four months I was gradually able to return to work – this was tough initially but provided a sense of balance and purpose for me going forward. Although it was tough knowing that a huge proportion of what I was earning was being spent on the divorce and the house I wasn't living in.

Another way of coping that was especially important to me was through creativity. I think that all creative people tend to have a lot to say after or during dark times, and that was certainly true for me, at least through my creative output. I actually wrote a book about everything that had happened to me – from getting sick all the way through recovery. This was my way of acknowledging that these things had actually happened to me, and I guess starting to work through them by putting them down on paper. It's still just a file on my computer for now, but maybe someday I'll pick it up again.

I also worked very hard on music – you have to remember I was effectively in lockdown for two years before the rest of the world, so I had a lot of time. Ultimately this meant that in the space of a year from 2019–2020 I released five albums on Blossöm Records, some of which directly addressed what I was going through at the time. I guess this was my version of 'art therapy'.

What have you learnt from your experience? And how therapeutic was your musical creativity?

I have learnt a huge amount from the last few years, both about myself and also other people. But perhaps the biggest takeaway ultimately has been just how incredible our bodies really are – healing from something so devastating obviously gives you a very specific perspective on this. I likened it at the time to the idea of being reset – what happened to me was essentially that I was turned off and turned back on again; and to go from not being able to move or walk, or eat, or go to the toilet alone – to then build myself back up and be able to run, swim, lift weights and become progressively stronger, faster and fitter. I have amazed myself at my resilience and inner strength. It has taught me to not be so hard on myself and to know that actually I'm doing OK.

At the time, I felt as if I had a deeper insight and understanding as to what was actually going on around us. It is very hard to explain, but my view of the world shifted. As I get further and further away from the experience, I feel myself getting further away from this insight, and I don't want to lose this – but all I have to do is to look at pictures from the time or read what I wrote – even writing this now, it's all still very fresh to me, and with that recollection comes that insight too.

On the flipside, it's made me (in some ways) less tolerant of people – who I can clearly see are not looking after their bodies. I would have no sympathy if you had a hangover for example! Our bodies truly are vessels, and we are all responsible for how we treat them. For some reason, huge amounts of people take this and their health for granted, and when it's nearly taken away from you, I think you have a responsibility then to go the other way as much as possible. There are many other learnings too, and I'm 99% sure that I wrote all about them in my book – that I haven't looked at in the last two years…

I have always throughout my adult life dealt with highly emotional events that have occurred to me through music. It is my way of dealing with these things and communicating them to the world. I don't know why, and in many ways, it would be far easier if I didn't – but this is the way I am wired. And so, creatively speaking, what happened to me resulted in five albums and an EP (extended play record) in the space of just over a year.

But perhaps more pragmatically than that, during the first year after I was ill, I was going through a prolonged and acrimonious divorce – that meant I had little money and a lot of time (the lockdown before lockdown) – and a lot of complicated feelings to deal with.

One of the albums appeared out of nowhere and was done very quickly in the space of about two weeks. I am old enough and have done this enough times by now, though, to realise that this is no coincidence, and that when something creative appears quickly, it is often the result of years' worth of subconscious work. But having that creative zone and vibe when I wasn't able to do much else was very inspiring and therapeutic – comforting almost.

I was very aware that I was doing something positive that would last forever (or at least all my life) with what had happened to me. My music is all instrumental, but I am describing what I went through very specifically on those albums. It's for the listener, of course, to interpret how they choose, but this is the place where they came from.

What advice would you give to someone else in a similar position to you?

Remember that your voice is ultimately the most important voice in your life. If something feels wrong, then it probably is. You have to listen to your gut – or guts in my case!

PART 5

Grieving, healing, therapy and personal change journeys

The recovery from traumatic and difficult challenges in life involves both grieving and healing.

Grieving and mourning for what has happened and what has been lost. Healing after the events towards a healthier future.

We can feel very alone at these difficult times. But what might help is to understand that you are not alone. Yes, your experiences are unique to you, but many others will, in their lifetimes, experience similar events that lead to grieving and mourning. While your journey is unique to your specific circumstances, there are stages of grief that have been experienced by millions of people.

One of these is explored in the next chapter. When you read through Elisabeth Kübler-Ross's description of the grief journey, you might be able to see how your experiences fit with her description. I have adapted her model to describe some typical reactions that might have been experienced as a result of the partial or full lockdowns that clamped down on personal mobility, social interactions and behaviours during the pandemic.

We then explore what happens when there has been a traumatic event in a person's life – one which interrupts a healing cycle. We then propose an approach that describes the road to recovery from trauma. Judith Herman contends that the central experiences of psychological trauma are disempowerment and disconnection from other people. Recovery then becomes based upon empowerment and the "creation of new connections". In her book *Trauma and Recovery: From Domestic Abuse to Political Terror*, Herman describes the stages of recovery as a healing relationship, safety, remembrance and mourning, reconnection and commonality.

Finally in this section, we explore how you can change on an individual basis. And it proposes that if you really want to change, then don't try to change! That might sound crazy, but it puts the emphasis on raising awareness as the precursor to change. This approach to change has been at the heart of my coaching style with clients for many years. And it worked for me on my recovery journey.

Chapter 30

The healing journey

By letting go of the old, we allow ourselves to the possibilities of the new.

Grief follows a course, but grief is unique to each individual. I learnt a few lessons from those occasions when family members and close friends have passed away.

- Firstly, their deaths have affected me very differently.
- Secondly, it is so difficult to 'fight' grief – it takes a lot of energy. Better to swim downstream and go with the flow than battle upstream.
- Time can feel grindingly slow, but time is a great healer.

Allow me to share a grief story, just two weeks after my father passed.

Case study

Keith's story

My father died many years ago in early December. He had been ill for some time, but his death came too quickly. I remember the time well because I was working away from home in the Docklands area of London. At the time I was publishing director of Golf World *magazine, which had just been acquired from its former US owners. It was a complex project, and I was very busy. The next few weeks were very hectic. Basing myself as much as possible with my mother, sorting out funeral arrangements and wanting to 'be there' for the family. Coupled with a very challenging time at work.*

On Christmas Eve, I travelled to my mother's house to spend Christmas with her. But I hadn't yet allowed my grieving process to start. I couldn't face just going straight to my mother's home from work. Instead, I went to the crematorium where his funeral had taken place and where his ashes were scattered.

It was the middle of the afternoon on a damp, freezing day. The ground was frosty, and snow was falling. It was growing dark, and I was the only visitor there. It was just me and a solitary member of staff who was on duty.

I walked round the grounds and let the grief flow. I couldn't stop the tears. In the end, daylight had faded to darkness, and there was just the illumination provided by the falling snow, the icy frozen paths and the distant lights from the crematorium building.

I got back into my car and headed for the exit – only to discover the gate had been locked and I was stuck inside. Not really the best place to spend Christmas, all things considered.

I returned to the main building and, fortunately, discovered that the man on duty hadn't yet left. He told me how to get out.

It left me thinking there was a message from my father – to take better care of myself and not to get locked inside the crematorium over Christmas.

Losing a loved one shifts the 'normal' and leaves a hole. It leads to a new and different paradigm. Just as, in its own way, the pandemic enforced a series of new normals, new paradigms. Life becomes different. Life is never quite the same again. I also believe that when people die, they don't 'go'. They are just out of sight.

My experiences of grief resonated with friends and colleagues coming to terms with their losses. On the one hand, people want to get on with their lives, but also handling the practical aspects of another's passing and allowing grief to take its course. Some try to fight it, but there is something about swimming down the river rather than trying to swim upstream. Grief will out, sooner or later.

We may well be overcome with grief at odd times. Sleep may be disturbed, or we might feel very vulnerable. And many people don't like to feel 'weak' or tired all the time. We can let ourselves heal and be kind to ourselves.

Perhaps we can progress at the pace that is appropriate for us; speaking with a therapist might also help. Allowing ourselves that duality of space to grieve, yet at the same time carrying on with the day-to-day of life. It can be a challenge to find that balance.

This is significant, especially with the many thousands of deaths from Covid-19. Far too many people were not allowed to say 'goodbye' to loved ones. The sheer brutality of the illness and then having to attend a funeral that was defined by physical separateness from even the closest family members.

What I experienced was grief, but it wasn't traumatic. Let's explore the journey for both of these.

What might the grief journey look like? We may feel alone in our grief, but the passage through grief is common to most of us. The model below, adapted from Elisabeth Kübler-Ross, provides a useful illustration to help understand – and make sense of – the journey through grief.

The journey through grief

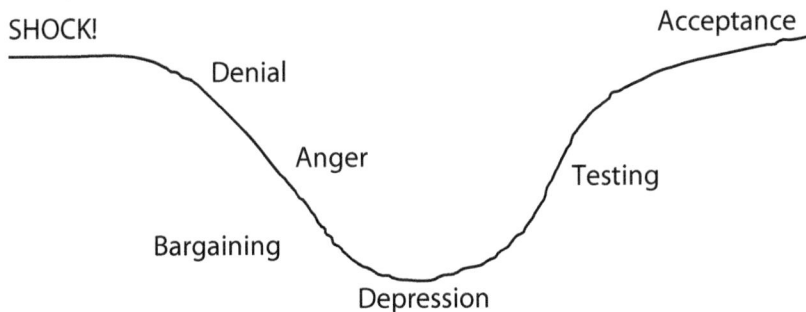

SHOCK!
Denial
Anger
Bargaining
Depression
Testing
Acceptance

Elisabeth Kübler-Ross originally described five stages of grief. Variations have since grown to seven stages that people go through. Here the different stages are considered within the context of national lockdowns. As you read through the stages, see if and how you can relate these stages to the lockdowns that you experienced – from announcement, to implementation, to living through it, to the easing down. Or perhaps if you were unfortunate enough to lose a loved one, you can relate your experiences to the model shown here.

The table below describes the stages of change and the types of responses that might be experienced at each step.

Stage of change	What we might experience
Shock	A shocked reaction to political leaders locking down many aspects of traditional living – especially in Western democracies, when freedoms were taken away.
Denial	The emotions you might have noticed were denial – "They can't close the pubs" and disbelief about what was going to happen. A great deal of shock, confusion and fears over the implications. For some people, their mood lifted: "It's about time they did something…"
Anger	The early stages after the change happened. There was a lot of frustration and anger at this time. Forced to stay at home. Not being able to go out. Lack of products on the supermarket shelves. There was a video that went viral of people fighting over toilet rolls in a supermarket. Moods dropped. Irritation. Perhaps anxieties were growing too.
Bargaining	Looking in vain for a way out, before acceptance.

Depression	This is the time of the real lows. We accept the inevitable. It's when we might have felt helpless, that it was never going to end. Perhaps when extensions to lockdowns were announced. It might have felt overwhelming. Seemingly no end in sight.
Testing	We explore new, realistic solutions. Maybe I could... Perhaps I might...
Acceptance	This is the time when we move on. We have accepted the change and find a way forward. Perhaps we decided working from home wasn't so bad after all. The commute to work was shortened from an hour to 10 seconds. We accepted the new reality. We transitioned through the stages. We saw new opportunities. Working from home might be preferable to the daily commute.

The grief journey can help to give shape to and make sense of our grieving and healing processes.

It's useful to see this as something that is not necessarily linear. Some people may return to previous stages of grief. (Just as some people may never come to terms with another's passing.)

The imposition of changes because of the pandemic was huge and immediate. These might have felt threatening and isolating. But although you might have felt alone, millions of people would have been going through their distinct – but resonant – personal journeys during the pandemic.

As ever, self-awareness is key. Notice your thoughts and emotions in the moment. The more you become aware, the better you can handle and respond to the changes. It may be tough, but generally greater self-awareness allows you to handle situations better, rather than them controlling you.

But what happens if we have been traumatized by the event? How does it compare with the grief journey? Perhaps it looks more like this:

The traumatic experience

SHOCK!

Normal self: a healthy self that carries on with life as normal

Survival self: coping with the ongoing legacy of trauma.

Prone to become traumatised self: experiencing memories of trauma as if in the present.

In the case of significant trauma, as above, there can be stuckness. Its level of suddenness and intrusiveness can be such that body and mind are both so shocked by the event that the person becomes locked down by the living legacy of trauma. There is a 'normal' or healthy self that carries on with life, but underneath this is the survival self, coping on a day-to-day basis and sometimes, for example, having flashbacks that bring the old trauma up into the present moment.

As we have seen earlier, some trauma is short-lived and recovery occurs after a few days, weeks or months. The illustration above highlights ongoing, unresolved trauma.

The chapters in this book explore ways of creating movement, of reducing the grip of trauma's legacy. In the next chapter, there is a model showing what the road to recovery from trauma might look like. It suggests a positive and sustainable way to move away from the position shown above.

CHAPTER 31

Discover your path on the trauma recovery journey

Recovery takes place with others.

One of the most courageous and significant steps you can take on your recovery journey is the decision to seek support and undergo therapy. It's a sad fact that many people are uncomfortable, anxious and afraid to look inside. They don't know what they might find. It can be difficult to trust others, including a therapist. Which means that they avoid it.

Yet over the last 20 years, there has been a tremendous growth in coaching. An increasing number of people have experienced some form of coaching at work in their professional lives, while there has also been a huge growth in the life coaching business.

You may have undertaken coaching and you may also have a valuable support network to help you – and there is so much that you can do to connect with others. A good coach will recognise their boundaries, and, if necessary, recommend or refer you to a therapist who will be professionally qualified and be in a better position to support you.

There are a number of factors to consider if you choose to work with a therapist:

- Firstly, their capability. The professional's capability to work with trauma – and perhaps specialized, specific trauma. They may also be able to work with (or link you with) specialised treatment if necessary, such as Eye Movement Desensitisation Reprocessing (EMDR).

- Secondly, the quality of the relationship. It is so important on the recovery journey.

I have benefitted from both therapists and coaches on my personal journey. They have helped in different ways, at different times.

Trust issues can be significant – both trusting yourself and trusting others. And, indeed, trusting yourself to trust others. If you've emerged from situations that leave you with low levels of trust, then putting your trust in someone else can be difficult. Those early meetings with the therapist can be experienced as challenging in different ways.

Connections with others are crucial. Working with an appropriate professional, and talking with supportive and empathic friends, are so helpful on this journey.

As I repeat throughout this book, what I write here in no way seeks to supplant therapy. My contention is that the book sits alongside such interventions and helps you on your individual journey through life. That progression from understanding, awareness and acceptance towards actions and new ways of doing and being.

There is a saying in Buddhism that when the student is ready, the master appears. There is your readiness to deal with the past and to start therapy. And in that therapy, a preparedness to explore, to open up. That readiness to open up within therapy might take many months.

A skilled and sensitive therapist will work with you appropriately, empathically, acceptingly and in a timely manner.

Trauma may be explored and revisited in ways that can be challenging and conducted in a manner that 'holds' you. So in this sense, you are working safely and being psychologically 'held' by the therapist. The trauma recovery journey can be shown like this:

The trauma recovery journey

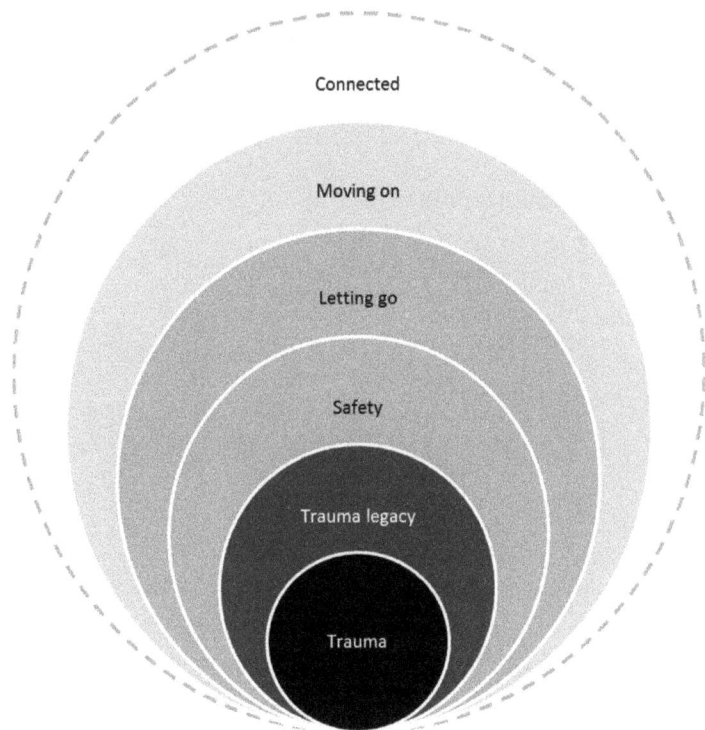

Making meaning from the model

Cover over the four outer circles, so that you can only see 'trauma' and 'trauma legacy'. That is the 'existing' reality, that might affect the traumatised person. Notice how dominant they become. Adding the additional circles open up so many opportunities for recovery.

These circles are designed with fluidity in mind. There may be a great deal of to and fro on this journey forwards and outwards. The trauma is often revisited, from ever-increasing distance.

As the circles widen, so the 'trauma' and 'trauma legacy' circles become proportionately smaller. They won't go away as they are a part of a person's history – but they are within a much more contained space. They have much less impact. They are much more manageable.

It echos the metaphor of the layers of an onion. But rather than just "peeling back" the layers, we are learning to look at the core traumatic event increasingly from this more distant, psychologically safe space: we can remember and mourn, but we can also bring ourselves back out safely.

The trauma recovery journey

Pre-recovery: living with trauma	
Traumatic event	Could be a single event; or repeated events; or multiple, complex traumas in different contexts. A single event could be just a few seconds, minutes or hours. Repeated trauma takes place over a prolonged period of time, perhaps over many years.
Trauma legacy	After trauma, getting on with life while coping with the after-effects. There is the 'mix' of the healthy self and the survival self – which struggles with the legacy of the trauma. Traumatic patterns occur. These can last a lifetime if unresolved. Effects can be passed on to future generations. People in this position often develop individual coping strategies. They might even make life-changing plans – and decisions – to choose to leave an unhealthy or abusive relationship. (Others use therapy first, and then decide to leave.)
The trauma recovery journey	
Safety ***(Understanding trauma)*** ***(Acceptance)***	Think of this as building a house. Safety creates the space for clearing the ground, working from the ground and digging down to lay and secure the foundations for recovery. Talking in a secure relationship helps to build this stable base. Behaviours that are healthy or counter-productive are explored. The self-care journey develops. There is a greater awareness of triggers that cause traumatic recurrences.

Letting go *(Grieving, healing and the change journey)*	The foundations continue to be embedded deep into the ground and the house building starts. Working through painful, traumatic memories in a way that is safe and 'held' psychologically, to remember and not recreate the trauma. This is a process that *relieves* the trauma, not *relives* the trauma. Exploring the past, experiencing grief, a sense of 'letting go'. Bringing to mind unremembered traumatic events. Mourning the past. Building understanding and awareness. The process of looking back can feel like being punched in the face. As memories emerge, these can feel painful – but there is a learning journey to roll with the punches. Over time, the punches become less severe.
Moving on *(Setting the scene to create your future)* *(Transform yourself)* *(Awareness into action)*	The house is being built and starts to take shape – with frequent checks back to the foundations. The walls go up and a roof is put on. This protects the building and allows development to be done on the inside. Remembering who you were; reconnecting, reinventing a sense of self and who you are. Creating a new, brighter future that is more empowered and builds new, supportive, trusting relationships. Increased ability to respond to traumtic triggers, rather than react (on autopilot) to them. Getting your needs met, taking action, increased self-care and clearer boundaries. Increased sense of power and control. Moving towards a brighter future.

Connected *(Live your best life)*	The house is complete and takes its place with the other houses. There are clear boundaries with the other houses, which together build a community. The foundations are solid, the walls and roof provide security and the inside is safe and compassionately furnished. The house is light and airy – a wonderful living space.
	There are doors and windows. Windows to see the world outside and allow the outside to see in. The doors can be left open and closed – and locked when appropriate. Window blinds can be opened and closed as a matter of choice. There is a sense of freshness, renewal, personal strength, stability and connectivity.
	The connections are noticeable through healthy relations with others and through a healthy, connected sense of self.

The recovery from trauma is very individual. It's your journey. The model is intended as an approximate and fluid guide.

Next, let's explore how change happens…

Chapter 32

How change happens

Why if you want to change, it might be helpful not to try to change.

Most people describe themselves as being comfortable with change. At a logical level, that makes sense! After all, I guess we don't like to be seen as the stick-in-the-muds who resist change.

At an emotional level, though, change can provide a bigger challenge. It's when the phrase 'resistance to change' is often heard.

Businesses like to talk about change and introducing change programmes. The business leaders then expect their co-workers to change, and quickly become concerned when they encounter resistance. For many people, their reaction to change is, first and foremost, what they might lose. That's hardly surprising. Often, they can't see any tangible benefits. Hence resistance. After all, why give something up which works well? As well as logical discussions around the costs and benefits of change, there can be emotional ones too.

There can be deeper resistance to change. Perhaps based upon beliefs or deeply buried memories from the past. Perhaps the result of previous challenging experiences that remain deep in the psyche. There is a concept called transference that plays out in our relationships. All our current relationships are coloured by our previous relationships. For example, the woman who had an abusive father might then find herself in relationships with a series of abusive partners. She leaves one, only to find the next. These themes of transference can be very impactful.

Resistance can be locked in at the physiological level when muscles have taken a protective and tight grip on the body. If you strain a tendon in your knee, for example, then expect your calves and thigh muscles to tighten up due to the additional, protective work they are doing. The challenge then is not only to repair the tendon, but also to ease back your calves and thighs to their more relaxed positions. It then seems these muscles need a lot of persuasion to loosen up, to let go of their protective stranglehold.

If our bodies have been locked down in some way by a traumatic experience, it may be a long process through awareness to recovery. Such strangleholds are not confined to our thoughts and feelings but held within the body. We will return to this theme later in this book and explore yoga later on. One way that you can help your body is to stretch these muscles and then breathe in and out within these stretches. This allows your body to start to 'acclimatise' within these stretched positions.

Sitting at the heart of recovery from traumatic experiences is change. Which often means making transitions at rational, emotional, gut and physiological levels. For people suffering with trauma, it can be particularly challenging – because the trauma can be so deeply imprinted in the body and mind.

And it's so often the case that people try to change, but their efforts to change don't achieve the desired outcomes. So what can be done to promote sustainable change?

Let's start with two words:

- Awareness.
- Responsibility.

Awareness is being aware of ourselves, our behaviours and our responses and interactions with others.

If we are unaware of our behaviours, are we likely to change them? No.

Yet if we become aware of our behaviours, we have a far greater potential for change.

Awareness grows through becoming more aware of ourselves. Our triggers, our biases, our filters. How we see ourselves, how we see others. How we relate with others.

From awareness comes responsibility. Response-ability, the ability to respond, the potential to make choices. We all have a choice: to do something or do nothing.

The two go together. Awareness leads to response-ability.

Yet how do you go about raising your awareness? And enhancing responsibility – your ability to respond?

In the context of change, there is a theory developed by Arnold Beisser. He called it the Paradoxical theory of change – which really is a bit of a mouthful, but it's a great concept to understand – and it correlates with the theme of awareness preceding and leading to response-ability. He wrote that *"change occurs when one becomes what he is, not when he tries to become what he is not."*

This is the paradox, according to Beisser. If we try to change (or if someone tries to change us), then we will not change. But if we stop trying to change and allow ourselves to become more aware of how we are now, then we can change.

I don't know about you, but when somebody tries to change me, I notice resistance within me. It feels as if I am being forced. It can seem that I am a problem to be fixed. Someone instructing me – *"Keith, you should…"* doesn't really get the reaction the other person might want or expect.

But how does Beisser's theory work in practice? Imagine you are a smoker and that you want to stop smoking. If you try to stop smoking, chances are you might not succeed.

His approach can be explained like this. Just become more aware of your smoking. You could keep a diary of your smoking 'triggers' that lead you to reach for a cigarette. Or become aware of the financial cost of smoking. If you smoke 20 cigarettes a day, that could cost you £13. Or £91 each week. Or getting on for £5,000 annually. You start to notice patterns. You become more aware of the impact it has upon you and others. Graphic images on packets are designed to raise this awareness. Then you might start to think differently. What else could you do with £5,000?

Perhaps his theory explains why so many new year's resolutions crash and burn too early into the next year – people are trying too hard to change.

So, rather than trying to change, focus instead on the here and now, enhance awareness, discover what's going on within yourself. Mentally, emotionally, physically. Raise your awareness. After all, awareness itself is curative.

This awareness gives us a greater ability to step into the future. If you've got a firm footing in the present – in your awareness of yourself – then you can step into the future. We literally need to ground ourselves in order to be in the position where we can move forwards. A firm footing in the present enables us to take those steps forward into our desired future. It's very difficult to step forward if your standing foot isn't firmly grounded.

Consider it as a combination of individual stability and an ability to move with the times. Isn't that what we are all trying to do? Not become "fixed" but to be able to move with the times, to ebb and flow as required.

The pandemic has challenged many "fixed" assumptions. Perhaps the art of prospering is to go with the flow, to be able to respond and adapt to a series of new 'normals' – and, through this, with a stronger sense of self.

Let's apply this theory to the trauma sufferer who wants to change, but time after time has found this seemingly impossible. And it is because the trauma was so rigidly imprinted within the body and mind that change was beyond his reach. Consequently, it becomes opportune to raise awareness instead.

Activity

Awareness-raising exercise

Consider a behaviour you wish to change. Allow yourself to become fully aware of it.

What is the behaviour you wish to change? Just focus on the present: how you behave in the moment. (Not how you want to change this behaviour, but how it is now.)

- What do you notice about it?
- How often does it happen?
- When does it happen?
- What triggers this behaviour?
- How much does it cost or impact you?

Allow yourself a few minutes to reflect upon these, without judgement.

This is a simple awareness-raising exercise. Once you have finished it, complete the box below.

What have I become aware of as a result of this exercise?

CHAPTER 33

Madeleine's story: escaping from 25 years of emotional abuse

Not all abuse is physical. Madeleine's story is that of emotional abuse, which built up during 25 years of marriage before she summoned up the courage to leave.

A combination of emotional abuse and coercive control is a heady mixture. It is different to physical abuse because the effects are not visible. Because you can't see the bruises, it is more difficult to identify and quantify than physical abuse.

Madeleine's story is, sadly, not that rare. I have met a number of Madeleines during my coaching journey. The cycle of abuse is used to help illuminate her story.

Escaping from 25 years of emotional abuse

Leaving a bad relationship can be so difficult. Abusive relationships are traumatic. Being abused in a relationship can feel isolating, demoralising and ultimately strip away self-belief and self-worth.

Have you heard the metaphor of the frog in the saucepan? If the frog leaps into hot water, it will jump straight out again. But if the frog is in cool, fresh water, it will relax. Over time, the water heats up until the time when the frog finds itself stuck in the boiling cauldron. Seemingly with no escape. Abusive relationships can leave the abusee in the same position as the trapped, overheated frog.

Watch the film *Gaslight* for how this works. The prospective partner who at first seems 'perfect'. So charming, so accommodating. Perhaps a whirlwind romance. And if someone appears 'perfect' – perhaps too perfect – then it might be best to be on your guard. In controlling and manipulative relationships, the word gaslighting refers to the controller's behaviour over the 'victim'. It leaves the 'victim' feeling a mixture of confusion, overly responsible, lonely, victimised, criticised, forever tiptoeing around eggshells and so on. She becomes confused and can lead to the recipient thinking that she might be going mad. [Men can also be victims.]

Abuse often follows a pattern, described as a cycle of abuse, shown below. If you are in an abusive, traumatic relationship, you might find yourself traumatised over and over and over again, mired in the sequences shown below. It follows a pattern with different phases – before, during and after an abusive outburst.

Cycle of abuse: the four stages of the abuse cycle

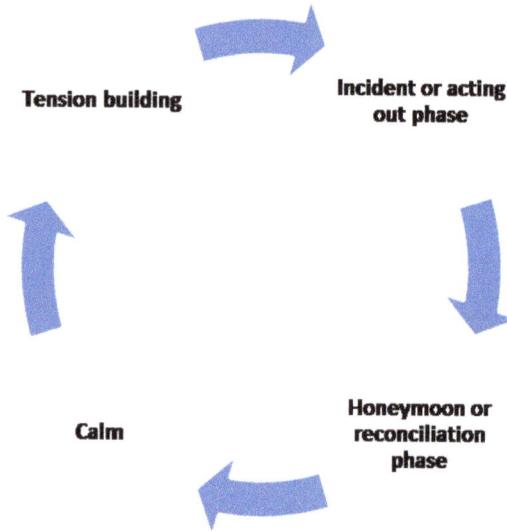

Tension building

Incident or acting out phase

Honeymoon or reconciliation phase

Calm

We will explore the abuse cycle in the context of Madeleine's experiences.

1) Tension building

The following behaviours are observed:

- Tension starts and steadily builds.
- Abuser starts to get angry.
- Communication breaks down.
- Victim feels the need to concede to the abuser.
- Tension becomes too much.
- Victim feels uneasy and a need to watch every move.

Madeleine writes:

This phase was like the guns on a battleship out at sea. It was like watching an old World War Two movie. I could see the ship's guns and, as I looked at them, would see them pointing forwards, always primed for action. Then the tension would build. Steadily and inexorably, the guns would swing around towards my direction. I knew that sooner or later (I never knew exactly when), they would be fired at me. I would become suffused with a sense of anxiety, uncertainty, dread and inevitability. Then the guns would be unleashed in my direction.

This process could be quite quick or could build over a period of a day or two. I could sense the anger. Nowadays I am very finely attuned to the merest hint of tension.

Sometimes I would know what the issue was, sometimes not. "What have I done?" This would be a recurring question in my mind. "Have I been so bad?"

Triggers in my husband would be:

- A "felt" perceived injustice. This was often the start point. If someone had done something to wrong him. He was great at becoming the victim.
- Somebody doing or saying something that pressed one of his buttons. So many inconsequential things. Mountains were made out of molehills. It was so easy for him to feel disrespected or threatened.
- Over-tiredness was another trigger.
- Threats to his level of control – for example over the finances, or our behaviours outside the home.

When two or more of these triggers combined, then the tension phase would be enhanced and much closer to the surface.

I would typically respond by:

- Seeking to keep things as normal as possible.
- Gently trying to reason without building the conflict.
- Deflect into safer areas. (Interestingly by asking him about his work, but this usually proved to be only temporary.)
- Walking on eggshells.
- Ensuring the children were on their best behaviour and would tiptoe around him.

My children also recognised this phase. My middle child (I have three) described the impact upon her as leaving her "pooping herself". She and my other children have discussed this, and both feared being the one who said or did the wrong thing and triggering their father's wrath.

2) Incident or acting out
- Any type of abuse occurs.
- Physical.
- Sexual.
- Emotional.
- Other forms, such as power and control.

Madeleine writes:

I describe the abuse as emotional and verbal. It has never been physical. Neither was it sexual.

My husband frequently described himself as having a tongue as sharp as a knife.

Outbursts were delivered with ferocious intensity. It was a monologue, a one-way conversation. I wouldn't describe this as an argument. (In my mind, an argument is a two-way interaction.)

Coping within this attack became a case of just taking it. I discovered the following responses to be unacceptable:

- *Silence: I was criticised for saying nothing.*
- *Trying to reason: It was not possible to reason with my husband when he was in this state.*
- *Arguing: This simply led to escalation and threats.*
  - *For me, the threat of him leaving. (I later realised this was one of his 'switches' to manipulate my behaviour.)*
  - *For my children, the threat of punishments and recriminations.*
  - *There was always an overt threat of further escalation and consequences.*

This was about power, domination and coercive control. He would not be challenged in this phase.

I nicknamed the venue for these outbursts as the "killing fields". For me, this was the bedroom. He would close the bedroom door and position himself in front of it. He would be standing; I would be sitting. I remember crying once, and he turned and walked away; such was his dominance. Sometimes the verbal attacks came in bed, in the dark in the middle of the night. I would wait for him to fall asleep. The car became another venue for the assaults. The pattern was always in a place of privacy, in a place of seemingly no escape, where I felt boxed in.

It lasted for as long as he decided.

I talked about it with my children after I had left. The eldest described the feeling as being "powerless". I would see my youngest daughter's eyes drop to the floor.

When I received this treatment, I felt trapped with nowhere to go. I just wanted it to come to an end.

It was like a raging river in full flood, sweeping everything in front of it and bringing a torrent of filthy, dirty, lingering water across the landscape. It left a devastating path of destruction and wreckage. In my metaphor for the event, the flood filled four houses (which represented me and the children). We were all still standing afterwards, but the residual damp would take a long time to dry out – if ever. He would then survey the scene afterwards, as if nothing had happened, apparently with no awareness of the devastation he had wrought.

Following these abusive tirades, I felt:

- *Exhausted.*
- *Relieved.*
- *Raging.*
- *Disempowered.*
- *Diminished.*

- *Psychologically punched.*
- *Grateful the storm had passed and hoping for calm again.*
- *I didn't want to be the one to break up the family.*

I don't do conflict well and wanted things to return to 'normal'.

His words cut through me like the knife he described. Some of the more memorable things he said and the threats he made were as follows. On one occasion when I threatened to leave, he told me that if I made a move for the door, then he would leave. He told me the reason he travelled so much was to get away from me. (He did have a number of affairs.) He told me that my texts were not nice enough. He also told me that I wasn't the woman I was when we first met. That's true, I was browbeaten.

In hindsight, I now see clearly the abuse, coercive control and elements of narcissism. Plus, of course, the ever-present manipulation. Looking back, the pattern followed key themes: the threat of 'consequences'; emotional manipulation (using the children to manipulate me), financial superiority and the need to be top dog.

One of the strange things that confused me was the 'switch' in mood. One moment he was raging at me or the children. Then he would stop, pick up the phone and become fully engaged and immersed in an upbeat conversation with work colleagues, friends or, as I later discovered, one of his 'flings'. I then realised this was not 'normal' behaviour. It left me bewildered and mystified. I could not switch from one mode to the next so immediately.

3) Honeymoon or reconciliation phase
- Abuser apologises for abuse; some beg forgiveness or show sorrow.
- Abuser may promise it will never happen again.
- Blames victim for provoking the abuse or denies abuse occurred.
- Minimising, denying or claiming the abuse wasn't as bad as victim claims.

Madeleine writes:

From my research on the internet, I always thought abusers apologised! This is one of the things that also confused me – and perhaps another reason for me not recognising this as abuse. He never apologised. He never said sorry.

He then twisted the responsibility – the perceived wrongdoing must be rectified. He would ask me:

"What are you going to do?"

He would ask this of whoever had supposedly 'wronged' him.

One conversation went like this:

Him: "What are you going to do (to improve)…"

Me: "I'm doing…"

Him: "That's not enough… I need to see more…"

He had a great skill in minimising the abuse as well, seeking to downplay his verbal violence.

The reconciliation phase in this family only started with the children's – or my – descriptions of what we would do. I just wanted to keep the peace, and unwittingly I became complicit in the abuse. I would say unwittingly as I hadn't brought into my awareness that it was abuse. It was only when I realised it was abusive that I decided to leave.

4) **Calm before the tension starts again**
   - Abuses slow or stop.
   - Abuser acts like the abuse never happened.
   - Promises made during honeymoon stage may be met.
   - Abuser may give gifts to victim.
   - Victim believes or wants to believe the abuse is over or the abuser will change.

Madeleine writes:

There is calm again. It was as if it never happened for him. For us, we deal as best we can with the emotional wreckage left behind by the flood waters. As I am discovering now, flooded houses take a very long time to dry out.

I hoped the shouting would go away, that the ripples in the pond would return to normal. But they never really did.

He would hand out gifts. I don't think he saw the irony of giving my youngest a electric scooter shortly after she was shouted at for not being at home enough. Luxury watches, opulent perfumes, the latest TVs, jewellery and much more besides.

But the gifts always came at a price. Me and the kids were repeatedly criticised. In hindsight it wasn't normal. Indulgent gifts and sharp criticisms were odd bedfellows.

When I left, I took nothing.

I have long thought that what I and the kids wanted weren't the monetary gifts but the emotional ones. Kindness, warmth, compassion and empathy.

For many years I hoped that we would live calmly moving forwards. I had been prepared to live with the outbursts because:

- *I wanted to keep the family together.*
- *One of the things I wanted most in life was a family.*
- *I was the family's caretaker.*
- *I doubted myself and my actions. Was it me causing the problems?*
- *It was only through counselling that I became more fully aware.*
- *I was in a hazy semi-awareness of the emotional abuse.*
- *I didn't want to be the wrecker.*

- *Through counselling, which started secretly long before I left, I discovered I had old and unresolved subconscious fears of abandonment.*

Madeleine describes her journey since leaving:

People have asked me why it took me so long to leave. Some even became frustrated with me. I just found it so difficult. I was extremely anxious; couldn't see a way out and was just afraid. I've since realised that taking a long time to leave is not unusual. It can take several attempts to break free. And many people end up returning to the abuser. As time went by, I developed my plans. It took a couple of years of therapy and planning before I made my escape.

A turning point was the day when my counsellor dropped in the word 'abuse' to describe what was going on. That day I cried more than I have ever cried before – or since. It validated my experience. I will never forget that day. Leaving the counselling room and driving more than half a mile up the road before I had to pull over and cry my eyes out. Yet it would take me another year to leave.

It's only since I left that I have realised more and more the depths of the coercive control, emotional abuse and manipulation – in so many different ways. The problem with emotional abuse and control is that the bruises aren't visible. They hurt inside. And from the outside, no one else sees what is going on. He was charming to others, the life and soul of the party. Nobody knew what went on behind closed doors.

He kept telling me that he loved me, but it felt like control. As far as I was concerned, it wasn't love. And I didn't love him. I don't think you can love someone you are afraid of. That fear ran deep. A word, a look or even a movement of the hand – any of those could traumatise me. It had become that bad.

I have as little as possible contact now. It's the way I can handle the situation and the necessary contact because of the kids. I also realised that contact could quickly grow out of control. Leaving him was, in his eyes, the ultimate betrayal. People who control don't like to let go. I keep contact to an absolute minimum.

I'm sure he had a lot of problems growing up as a child, which makes it very sad. But he's an adult now and has to take responsibility for his words and behaviours. And I do too. And I don't want that in my life anymore.

Now I can rest and relax peacefully and, day by day, build my new life. The healing process is wonderful.

Leaving was the toughest thing I have ever done in my life. Behind having children, it was the best thing I did in my life. I realised I am a survivor.

Life is very different now. I am not shouted at and I feel much freer. I sleep more peacefully at night now. And that's truly wonderful.

PART 6

Setting the scene to create your future

This is the shortest section in the book.

It involves action – and action requires a single first step.

What might seem psychologically significant can be, paradoxically, very simple.

Creating your future starts with a single step.

Chapter 34

Create your future

It's up to you to see and move towards future possibilities.

The future is any moment in time that has yet to happen. It could be an hour away or a day or a week away. Maybe a year or a decade. Or even longer.

Eventually the future will become the present, and then become the past.

What is your relationship with the future?

Many 'experts' and coaching books encourage you to set goals for your future. And that is great. But not for everyone. It is too simplistic.

Some people find it easy to set goals, others don't. Through many coaching sessions, I have asked clients what goals they might want. For some, these come relatively easy, and they set short, medium, and long-term goals. They have a clear outcome in mind and can then plan accordingly.

For others, however, they simply do not think this way. The concept of setting long-term goals seems like speaking a foreign language to them. In coaching, asking them to think about the long term feels like swimming upstream. The client doesn't get very far, it is hard work, and the energy level drops. (And it is perhaps difficult to set goals if the client is still dealing with unresolved issues from the past.)

In these cases, we can take it a step at a time. Small steps to create movement. Stepping from the present into the future. For the individual dealing with unfinished business, creating that sense of a future may feel difficult. It can feel somewhere too far beyond the horizon and quickly bring on feelings of helplessness. A useful time to remember that a journey of a thousand miles starts with a single step.

That single step, however seemingly small, can be crucial.

Case history

Olivia's story

Olivia held a director level position in a major London business. Single, she had fallen into the habit of working late at work every day and getting home tired each evening, sometime after 7 o'clock. As she spoke, it was clear her energy levels were very low.

I asked her what she liked to do when she wasn't working. She thought about it and replied, "Ceroc dancing." I asked her when she last went dancing. She told me that she hadn't been dancing for over six months. She had fallen out of the habit and was too tired to go once she was home. Coincidentally, she told me, there was a Ceroc class that evening.

Her single action from the coaching session was to leave work promptly, get home and then attend the dance class.

That simple, single action had a significant impact for her.

She had disconnected from that part of herself that took a lot of pleasure, energy and meaning from dancing. Reconnecting allowed her greater integration within herself. Becoming more whole in this way allowed her to reconnect with her energy that seemed to have drifted away. She had started to move – in a very energetic way. Ceroc replaced the sofa.

Getting back in touch with her energy had a huge impact at work. Having renewed her personal sense of energy, she was promoted shortly afterwards.

Creating your future

I invite you to complete **either** or **both** of the exercises below, depending upon your relationship with goals.

Do remember this too:

How you behave today will create your future.

I have coached many people who are extremely busy in their lives. Sometimes, at work, I think it is difficult to distinguish between 'business' and 'busyness'.

Today they are busy, and tomorrow they want to be more relaxed. But when tomorrow comes, they are just as busy tomorrow as they are today. They are well and truly on the hamster wheel.

Their past was busy, their present is busy, and their future will, in all probability, be busy. Driving themselves hard, afraid, and sometimes not able to see a way out.

And tomorrow becomes next week. Next week becomes next month. Next month becomes next year. Next year becomes next decade. Still on that same old hamster wheel. Then they die. They've got more than enough time on their hands then. My recommendation is that you don't allow yourself to be that person, unless it's what you really want.

Remember, how you behave today will play a huge role in leading you into your future. And you always have a choice. Remember, the key is in your pocket.

Activity

Goals, taking steps and creating movement.

You may or may not be able to describe goals. Feel free to complete the exercise below as best suits you. If you find it difficult to complete (1) Setting goals, then move on to sections (2) and (3).

1. **Setting goals**
   Think of up to three long-term goals you might have. If there is only one, that's fine.

Goal	What will be a great outcome?	When will this be achieved by?

2. **First steps**
   Identify up to three small steps that you might take that would create movement within you. This could be something new or different you would like to do.

First step	How this will benefit you

3. **One thing you could – and will – do differently towards achieving your goals and creating movement within you**

Activity

Write your headline!

Imagine you are writing a headline for yourself sometime in the future. The timing is up to you. The headline celebrates a fantastic outcome for you. Write the headline in the space below. And write a date for when you will have achieved this headline.

Date:

CHAPTER 35

John's story: from the battlefields of war to the offices in England

John is a friend of mine who is one of those people who cannot do enough for others. Courteous, considerate and professional, you could easily describe him as an officer and a gentleman. Well, former officer to be precise, because he left the military and now works in private enterprise. Before I write more about him, please allow me the indulgence of replaying a quote from the film *The Bourne Identity* where the main character, Jason, is sitting in a café and tells his companion that he can recall the numbers on the licence plates on the cars in the car park, has seen that the waitress is left-handed and can estimate the weight of a customer sitting by the counter.

John possesses that type of vigilance. On one occasion, when I met him for a meeting in a London hotel, I was struck by how aware he was of his surroundings. He had located the optimum seats for our private conversation. The seat had its back to the wall and was tucked away in a far corner. As someone who regularly has meetings in hotel lobbies, I take pride in finding somewhere private to sit but hadn't even seen that discreet location. It told me how alert John is and how much he notices.

Many years of active service in a successful military career had heightened John's awareness of his surroundings. Yet his awareness, and his considerateness for others, didn't prevent his transition from military to civilian work from passing without disturbance. Today he has successfully completed this transition, but on the way was diagnosed with, and has successfully put behind him, the traumas he experienced on his journey.

The questions in the account that follows are ones I put to him. Here's John's story…

John's story: from military to civilian life

Please give me an overview of the traumatic event – what happened.

I joined the military in the 1990s and put my time and effort into being the best I could be. That mantra stuck with me for many years, and I ended up serving for 20 years. I was promoted rapidly and did very well in all aspects of my career.

As life evolved, I met and married my wife, and we travelled the world together. In time, we had two children, and the military way of life started to become more difficult with a growing family. We decided that it was time for me to leave the military, a choice that seemed fairly easy to make at the time.

I was allowed to leave the military quite quickly. There was an ongoing redundancy programme to shrink the size of the UK's armed forces, and although I was not able to take advantage of the redundancy, I was able to leave more quickly than normal. The result was that from resigning to actually leaving took less than three months, a resettlement programme that would ordinarily be spread over a year. The resettlement process is designed to transition service personnel from service life to that of the 'ordinary' world, something that I didn't have, and most importantly until now, didn't realise that I needed.

The trauma that I began to experience came from the memories and flashbacks from a combination of high-intensity operations in Bosnia, Iraq, Sierra Leone and Afghanistan, combined with a feeling of self-loathing [I later discovered that I was upset with others, but took responsibility and internalised the blame] and separation anxiety caused by the rapid change from my military career to the civilian world. The departure from the military and a rapid transition from one career to another was more significant than I had ever envisaged through my thought process of deciding to resign from the military.

I began to have sleepless nights, anxiety and severe imposter syndrome. These alone would have been bad enough, but alongside these issues were troubles in my new civilian employment. Working in a civilian environment was very different to that of the military. It ended up in us parting company. At the time, it felt life-ending, with no clear vision to be able to support my partner and children and a re-ignition of the feelings of self-loathing.

The military provides a comforting, cosseting place that creates a unique environment for service personnel to do their jobs in the most effective way. This is a necessary part of the military way of life but needs a period of readjustment when moving to civilian life and working.

I missed that period of adjustment, moving from high-intensity military operations in Afghanistan, Iraq, Africa and other places in the world, entering another profession where I had to quickly come to terms with new ways of working, a different language and quite uniquely, a situation in which I discovered that the meaning of integrity is very different. The military ingrain in all service personnel the Values and Standards, which is something that I still hold true today but recognising that these 'rules' are not part of everyday civilian life made things hard for me. The Army leadership code described this distinctness from society at large:

> "The Army Leadership Code is founded on our Values. To us, Courage, Discipline, Respect for Others, Integrity, Loyalty and Selfless Commitment are much more than words on a page, they are what the British Army stands for, and what sets us apart from society."

My personal life remained very good, with my partner and children supportive of what I was doing in my new professional life, together with a decent home, health, and happiness. But with difficulty in finding acceptance in my new job, I began to struggle with things. Relationships were more complex and problematic within the work culture that I experienced. This became the sticking point, and the effect on me was profound, causing me to have sleepless nights, feeling worthless, and flashbacks to the most significant moments in my military career.

In the early days of this, I did do not very well. I only recognised what was happening to me when a good friend explained that I probably needed some help. I was tired and not in a great place, and this was showing in my mood and general attitude.

Things were so bad that I ended up being placed under the care of a leading trauma psychologist, who helped me over a period of months to understand what was happening to me and how I could cope with the feelings and thoughts that invaded my mind on an hourly basis. This medical help was for the things that I had experienced in the military but also the new pressures created from my new choice of profession.

It wasn't long before I was diagnosed with Post Traumatic Stress Disorder (PTSD), and whilst the diagnosis was only mild in nature, it was nonetheless something that we could all work on solving.

The worst part was being in the middle of a mental maelstrom but not recognising it, with pressure on my family and me from both historic and present-day issues.

I eventually decided that it would be right for me to leave my job, and in hindsight can see the scale of the challenges from transitioning from a military to a civilian working life. This all took a tremendous toll on my physical and mental health, causing higher than normal levels of anxiety and worry from the thought of a loss of income and perhaps losing our family home.

I spent time reflecting on what had happened, the causes and what I needed to do to move forward. I was lucky to have had the opportunity of some coaching training that allowed me to be introspective and think about how my life had developed since leaving the military.

The trauma counselling also helped, allowing me to recognise that the experiences I had endured in my time in service were not my fault. This gave me the space to breathe and look to the future. I also had a wonderful family who supported and guided me through this dark time, giving me support and space to reflect and grow.

Moving forwards was not as daunting as I expected. The jump that I thought would be necessary was actually a small step, something that I consider to be very lucky.

I spent my time looking for a new job and volunteering in the local community, both of which allowed me to slow the pace of life and be very reflective and deliberate about each decision I was making. Looking for a new job was another anxious time, but I was lucky to remain with my employer through to finding a new job, with the transition from old employer to new taking place over a weekend. Although those weeks leading up to leaving my old job were some of the longest in my life, I found myself working in a new company with friendly colleagues and a bright future.

When you look back on these events from a distance, were there other ways in which you were able to strengthen yourself?

The strength that came from knowing that I had support was the main thing that kept me sane. I was also fortunate enough to be physically active and live in the countryside, so long walks with my wife and dog, along with getting physical exercise through running, were all beneficial to my mental state of mind.

What advice would you give to someone making the transition from military to civilian working and living?

Take your time! The transition is much more difficult than you will ever imagine, and so researching the right role for you and taking advice are also both crucial to making sure that your second career is as successful as possible, right from the outset.

What advice would you give to someone living through PTSD?

I don't feel as though the label of PTSD is something that I deserve. I have friends and colleagues who have 'real' or more serious PTSD, and even now the diagnosis makes me uncomfortable.

However, the key to any form of stress, anxiety or mental health issues is to recognise that you need help and seek out the support and help that you need. The main thing for me was being able to recognise my triggers and to deal with them as they occurred, speaking with my coach, the doctor and my friends and family.

PART 7

Transform yourself: being and becoming

This is the first of three sections in this book that focus on practical and achievable approaches that you can integrate within your developmental journey.

Being and becoming encourages you to think about how you 'are' – the being – and how that can be used towards becoming – becoming the person that you want to be.

Subsequent sections focus on practical activities that you can do.

These sections are deeply interconnected. Their purpose is to demonstrate how your way of being – coupled with what you can do – can be combined to help your transformation. These two aspects – being and doing – are deeply interconnected and lead to becoming.

- Now is a time to look back less and to look forward more.
- Now is a time to unhook the chains from the past and take off into a brighter future.
- Having accepted the past is over, now is a time to look forward with greater confidence and belief.

CHAPTER 36

The journey of being and becoming who you want to be

It's better to show up fully in the here and now than continually grapple with your past.

Doing, being, becoming, learning. These four words sit at the heart of the journey of being and who you want to become.

The focus here is upon being. Take a pause to consider your life and how you live it. Here are a few questions to think about.

- When you are preparing a meal, are you putting something in the microwave or taking time to prepare a meal with freshly cooked ingredients? (Think about this particularly in the context of cooking for yourself and/or cooking for others.)
- If you have a home with a garden, do you see the garden as a chore or something that is – or can become – a beautiful living space?
- If you exercise, do you see it as a should-do activity to try to keep fit or as an opportunity to create a fitter, healthier and more vibrant you?

Perhaps you fall partly into both camps. There are many more examples we can think of. During the early stages of the first 2020 lockdown, I was shocked to see the number of people piling into tube trains in London. At that stage, not wearing masks, and pressed up against others. I am sure a considerable number of people made those journeys out of necessity, but I wonder what proportion of those passengers might have travelled at a different time, or walked, or cycled. To what degree were they practising self-care, I wonder.

In life, we can always just 'do', or perhaps we can make a choice to allow ourselves to 'be'.

Think about the prison population for a moment. There is a particular phrase that is used – prisoners 'do' time in jail. A convict is 'doing' 10 years for his crime. Prisoners are confined behind locked doors, enclosed in cells and have a lack of freedom. It makes me wonder what prisons we create in our own minds. If we are just 'doing', then maybe we are experiencing our own life sentences. Maybe we are just doing our own time.

Of course, there are many things we *have* to 'do' in life – it can't always be a peak or 'in the zone' experience. But perhaps we can ensure it is more meaningful, with a greater sense of purpose.

There is the often-repeated story of the three people working on a building site. A passer-by asks the three people what they are doing.

- The first replies: "I am laying bricks."
- The second replies: "I am building a wall."
- The third replies: "I am creating a beautiful home."

If you think about the building site that is your life and you were asked this question, what would your answer be?

Have you ever paused to consider the following questions?

- What motivates you?
- What do you value?
- What gives you meaning?
- What is your purpose?

Questions such as these offer the opportunity to expand our life's experiences from just doing to a more meaningful 'being'. Many years ago, I edited various magazines. One of the most memorable was *Trail* magazine – which I created and launched onto the market in 1990. It is still available today.

Its purpose was to enrich the lives and experiences of people who love long-distance walking in remote places.

While the sales team was focused on revenues and the publisher was interested in profit, my aim was simple. To create a wonderful magazine that would resonate with readers. If I could do that, and enrich the lives of sufficient numbers of people, then revenues and profits would follow. It was a simple philosophy. And I had a second purpose too. To create new magazines and products that would generate more jobs for people. So that job provided both meaning and purpose and was a very successful and memorable time in my career. It provided me with great energy and focus. It was a case of discovering and continually finding the 'sweet spot' with readers.

And that's what your journey is about – for you to discover your 'sweet spots' – where you are energised, feel comfortable, and allow yourself to grow through how you are and what you do.

We can look at our lives in terms of doing, learning, being and becoming, which I have adapted here:

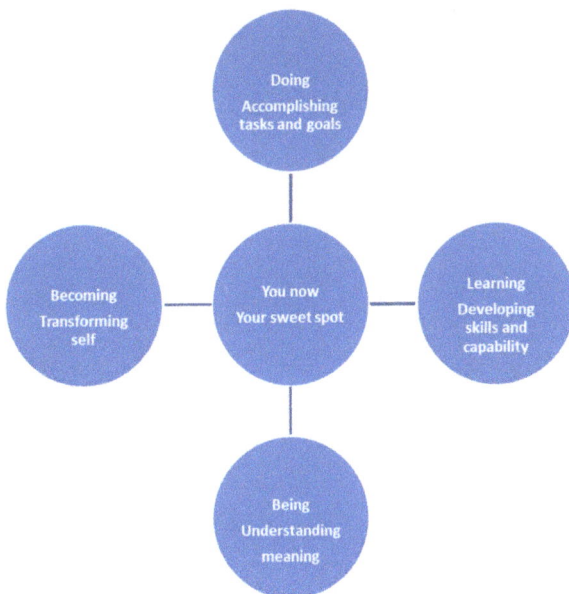

Consider your life right now.

Doing: to what degree are you achieving tasks and goals? Or are you just 'going through the motions'?

Learning: what are you continuing to learn as you progress through your life?

Being: what meaning and fulfilment are you experiencing, even (perhaps especially) in so-called 'simple' tasks?

Becoming: who are you becoming? Who might you become? What opportunities are you creating for your transformation of self?

Sunny Stout-Rostron links two of these together: being and being-in-becoming. If we can really allow ourselves to 'be' in the moment – if we enrich our being, then who might we become? This is the transformation of self. This is when people who are burdened by the past might step into a much freer, self-created present and future. This time is now: when you can leave behind the burdens of the past and step forward from the here and now into the future: more intimately, autonomously and spontaneously.

Your opportunity is now. And by now, you know where the key is!

CHAPTER 37

Rethinking and resetting post-traumatic stress disorder to include post-traumatic growth

Let's hear it for post-traumatic growth!

While post-traumatic stress (PTS) and post-traumatic stress disorder (PTSD) have widely entered everyday language, post-traumatic growth (PTG) is heard much less frequently. Yet it is important to consider trauma from this perspective too.

The qualities often described within PTG include:

- Growing personal strength; developing new resilience.
- Enhancing your relationships with others.
- Enjoying a deeper appreciation of life.
- Benefitting from spiritual growth.
- Identifying and seeking out new possibilities.

Let's look at these five domains in turn.

	New possibilities open to you
	Greater appreciation of life around you
Five domains of PTG	Your personal strengths and qualities
	Your close relationships that are appropriate for you
	Your personal growth and development

Personal strength

This is an optimistic position that says, "I can." It is built upon resilience and resourcefulness. An increased capacity to meet life's challenges. Words such as self-reliance, wisdom and personal qualities all spring to mind. An overall sense of personal capability and capacity.

Relationships with others

The ability to build and then sustain close, intimate relationships. Being able to distinguish between those people with whom you can safely connect and those with whom you do not wish to become closer. Reaching out to others and recognising both parties' needs and wants. Building a sense of loving and allowing yourself – and the other – to be emotionally vulnerable, safely. Accepting you need contact with others. Allowing yourself to swim in the stream of life with others. And letting go and walking away from those relationships that do not add value to you or may detract from you and your journey.

Spiritual development

Personal growth and development – whether described by one person as spiritual development or another as mindfulness. Finding a greater meaning and purpose in life. Meditation. More deeply philosophical.

New possibilities

Just because one of life's doors has slammed shut in your face doesn't mean that there aren't other doors. The footballer or ballet dancer's careers that have been shattered through injuries don't prevent those individuals from pursuing careers away from their initial chosen fields. New interests, new perspectives, experimentation, discovering and exploring new possibilities. Not allowing yourself to be defined by your past trauma and other challenging experiences. Letting go of the old to allow in the new.

Greater appreciation of life

An overall greater appreciation of life. Acceptance. Working out what is important in life. Enjoying the small things. Redefining your priorities and discovering new ones. Working from home during lockdown has had a transformative effect on many people. Rediscovering close family relationships and not spending laborious hours travelling to and from work every day. Appreciating daily walks and bike rides with the family.

Case study

Keith's story

"My response to dealing with trauma consisted of both PTSD and PTG – although I didn't fully appreciate the latter for many years. Subconsciously, my life was both in survival mode (PTSD) and coping/ thriving (PTG). This came to the fore when I was editing a magazine and needed to radically change its format. I was told I would never achieve my goal, but I did. Whenever people told me I couldn't do something, then it was like a red rag to a bull – I used their negativity as a motivator for me. Some things took an awful lot of courage.

I experienced this while editing a magazine called Athletics Weekly. *I am a passionate believer in 'fair' competition, and before taking on the role, thought that drug-taking in the sport was not a problem in the UK. I remember talking with the then president of the European Athletic Association, Sir Arthur Gold, who was an uncompromising enemy of drug-taking. His challenge was one of proving a case against the drug cheats – as he believed (as I do) that they should have lifetime bans. He told me that at UK events, if an athlete (who he knew was a drug-taker, but could not prove it) won an event, he would sit with his arms crossed, not applauding the athlete.*

As editor of the magazine, I championed the fight. In one issue, I dispensed with a picture of an athlete on the front cover (for the first time in the magazine's 40+ year history) and ran different drug-related stories inside. These included an (anonymised) interview with an English athlete who was regularly taking drugs, wiring up a journalist who easily bought steroids from a gym in Essex and breaking a story in the UK of a German athlete, Birgit Dressel, who took steroids and died from multiple organ failure, aged just 26.

Choosing this course of action was personally alarming. Perhaps it's easiest to say that I received a lot of cold shoulders while I remained in that job! It felt like being a 'whistle-blower'. And this was a year before Ben Johnson tested positive at the Seoul Olympics.

My PTG was taking the fight forwards against cheating. My PTSD, coupled with the reaction from others, was alarming and isolating. It was not an easy time. Would I do the same again? Absolutely I would.

In more humble surroundings, I noticed I would also do things in my way. In team meetings, I often seemed to be the individual throwing in the curved ball. Or coming up with a left-field suggestion that was either accepted with appreciation or fell on deaf ears. I wasn't too bothered either way, but I did seem to exist on a different planet at times.

I achieved in work – if I needed to stay late, I did. I worked very hard, resiliently and creatively. I owned my outcomes.

At the same time, I paid a price for this. I struggled with relationships; my lack of self-belief drove me harder. And I wasn't prepared to let my career stagnate. I changed jobs, moved companies, and reinvented my career, eventually working for myself.

It was while working as a coach that I discovered my purpose in life – to help people lead their lives in richer and more fulfilling ways – and spent many years focusing on personal growth and development to get a greater sense of meaning in my life too. The more I could achieve that, the better I could help others.

My life was a mix of two things. Part survive, part thrive. I was aware of this duality in my life. The successful life and the struggling life. Becoming a coach was transformational. Huge amounts of self-development and self-growth deepened my levels of self-awareness, enhanced my self-regard and restored my self-belief – crucial to supporting others.

I've now reached the stage in my life where I have been able to work through traumatic memories and focus on the PTG. But it has been a long journey.

Perhaps one of the greatest learning points for me has been this duality – this capacity to hold both 'disorder' and 'growth' simultaneously. People who have had traumatic experiences remember the horrors, but also can recognise the inner responses of surviving, coping and, basically just getting on with life. They often don't realise (or dismiss) the fact that they have become extremely adept and resilient. They may even just simply experience PTG. As Nietzsche said, 'That which does not kill us, makes us stronger'."

Activity

Explore your personal PTG domains

Use the table below to reflect upon your personal PTG domains. In the centre column, note down your thoughts on where you are now. In the right-hand column, consider and explore what opportunities might lie ahead for you.

Domain	Your thoughts on this domain as it applies to you	Your opportunities to grow your personal strength
Personal strength The optimistic position that says, "I can."		

Relationships with others Ability to build and then sustain close, intimate relationships.		
Spiritual development Finding a greater meaning and purpose in life, whether 'spiritual' or mindfulness.		
New possibilities New interests, new perspectives, experimentation and trying out and discovering new possibilities.		
Greater appreciation of life Acceptance. Working out what is important in life. Enjoying the small things. Redefining your priorities and discovering new ones.		

CHAPTER 38

65 affirmations to boost your confidence

Many of us talk to ourselves, so let's make sure it's constructive and positive!

Affirmations provide wonderful self-talk. They are simple, clear and unequivocal sentences you can say about yourself and to yourself. Repeatedly.

Read through the list below. Some of these affirmations may resonate with you, others may not. You can develop a set for yourself. Or you may want to create your bespoke affirmations. You can find many on the internet.

It helps to establish these as constant reminders. You might want to set an affirmation as a screensaver, post it on your fridge door or bathroom mirror, or pop it in your wallet or purse. Perhaps you could write it on a postcard – and occasionally send it to yourself!

Do see if you can read your affirmations several times daily. Say an affirmation out loud while you are getting yourself ready for the day. Keep repeating these affirmations, day after day. Affirm to yourself to get into the affirmation habit!

And remember. These are very quick and easy wins and a chance to give yourself some precise, accurate and positive self-talk!

1. I am a competent and confident person.
2. I learn from my mistakes and those of others.
3. I am an attractive and interesting person.
4. People listen to what I have to say.

5. I am persuasive and influential.
6. I am responsible for myself and my actions.
7. I am independent of the approval of others.
8. I can always find opportunities in situations of change.
9. I am creating my desired future.
10. I am what I am.
11. I have all the resources to do what I want to do.
12. I am at one with myself and my world.
13. I am free to be what I want to be.
14. I respect myself and all living things.
15. In loving myself, I love others.
16. I am continually developing my inner self.
17. All things have meaning, and there is always opportunity in adversity.
18. In giving, I achieve more.
19. I am open to the opportunities this day brings.
20. I am in control of my thoughts, my words, and my life.
21. My courage is stronger than my fear.
22. I trust myself to make the right decisions for me.
23. I have the ability to create the life I desire.
24. I do not allow my past to control my future.
25. I am important.
26. My life is meaningful.
27. I matter.
28. I am capable of transforming negative experiences into something positive.
29. I am worthy of respect and equality.
30. Everything will work out for my highest good.
31. I learn to love myself unconditionally, more and more every day.
32. I am opening my heart and learning to trust again.
33. I know my truth.
34. I feel anxious, and I know what that feels like, and I'll get through it.
35. All my emotions are legitimate. I let myself be happy, sad, frustrated and hurt. This is my experience, and I am accepting it.

36. Each day, I am creating a more meaningful life.
37. I am changing in positive ways. I am making peace with my past and accepting myself.
38. I am safe when I'm near other people.
39. I make healthy choices and choose to love myself a bit more every day.
40. I am exactly where I need to be on my journey.
41. I am strong, independent and respect my boundaries.
42. I am safe.
43. I see every situation as an opportunity to heal and grow.
44. I choose to focus on the things I can control.
45. My needs and wants are just as important as anyone else's.
46. Everyone has something to teach me, I rise above the events and see the bigger picture.
47. I trust my instincts and listen to my inner wisdom.
48. I am excited to start a new page in my life.
49. I am OK.
50. I am who I am, and that is fine.
51. I allow my true self to flourish.
52. I believe in myself and my abilities.
53. The past is over, and it has no power over me now. I refuse to be a victim anymore. I claim my power.
54. I am who I want to be.
55. My body is getting stronger each day.
56. I let go of my feelings of pain and let come in feelings of loving kindness for myself.
57. I inhale strength and exhale fear. I am learning that it is safe for me to heal and grow.
58. I have the ability to create the life I desire.
59. I choose to live my life to the fullest.
60. I deserve to be loved.
61. I deserve to be respected.
62. I have the power to change my story.
63. I do not allow my past to control my future.
64. I choose to let go of the past and look forward to the good that awaits me.
65. As I forgive myself, it becomes easier to forgive others.

Activity: your affirmations

Having read through the list, what are the affirmations that resonate most with you? Use the table below for noting down your top three affirmations. Or you might want to create your own affirmations. The choice is yours. Like so many other things in life, it's up to you.

Tip: if you create your own affirmations, then do the following:

- Own the affirmation. Start the affirmation with "I" or "My".
- Write the affirmation in the present tense.

My affirmations

CHAPTER 39

Attend to your felt sense

Notice and acknowledge your inner self, both body and mind.

Eugene Gendlin first coined the phrase "felt sense" back in 1978. Your felt sense isn't something you experience mentally. Neither does it pop into your mind through words or thoughts. It's a bodily sensation, a bodily feeling. And it's more than emotions – a combination of emotional and factual components that are contained within your body. The challenge is that it might not be apparently evident to us as we go through our daily lives. He described it as "a kind of body awareness that profoundly influences our lives and that can help us reach personal goals."

One way to start to think about felt sense is how you might describe another person. Let's just say that you had been flying away on holiday and, waiting in the airport lounge, you bumped into – and struck up a conversation with – someone famous. If you are telling a friend about your encounter with this well-known person, often the first question your friend might ask is:

"What is she/he like?"

A factual reply might describe the clothes they were wearing, the colour of their shoes, distinctive facial features, what they were carrying and so on. But who answers in that way?

The questioner wants to get a sense of what they are "really" like in terms of a "felt sense". And that is often a main factor in your reply. If you reply:

"She's very friendly – she even bought me a cup of tea," then you are, in some way, talking from your felt sense – that you were struck by her friendliness that created a warm sensation within you.

Contrast it with:

"He was a bit creepy – he sat very close to me, and I could smell alcohol on his breath."

Here there is a felt sense of intrusion and a dis-ease that made you want to get away from his company. It is part factual, part emotional, but reflective of your interpretation of that individual. And notice how the felt sense picks up on both the holistic aspect (whole person) and some specific details too.

The felt sense described here is a response to another person. It can also be a response to your environment and, crucially, to yourself. Let's see how it might apply to you.

I remember talking with a couple of elderly people in their 70s. Brother and sister, they were reminiscing about childhood memories – specifically watercress and stilton cheese sandwiches they used to eat during the family tea on Sunday afternoons. It brought back pleasurable memories of simple, happy, family times from many years earlier. A strong, warm, remembered felt sense. Relating this story here gives me a warm, comfortable feeling in my stomach.

How do you become more aware of your felt sense? The good news is that, over time, you can become more aware of and in touch with your felt sense.

One way to start is with an event that has pressed a trigger within you. Let's explore this through a case study to see how it unfolds.

Case study

Fiona's story

I was coaching Fiona, who worked for an organisation with 300 employees. She had been promoted from head of finance to financial director. With that promotion came a place on the male-dominated board. Part of the purpose of the coaching was to support her journey towards taking an active role in board meetings. Through the coaching discussion, we had reached the place where she had shared her anxieties around attending the meeting with a group of suit-wearing male executives, some of whom she described as being of the alpha male variety. She had recently attended her first board meeting.

Keith: How was it for you to attend the board meeting?

Fiona: It was OK. I felt quite nervous, but at the start the CEO welcomed me to the meeting, and everyone congratulated me. But it felt like a honeymoon period. After that, the meeting became quite feisty. The third quarter hasn't been good, and sales have been poor.

Keith: What happened?

Fiona: There was a lot of tension between sales and production. Mike, the sales director, can be aggressive and blamed Carlos, who got very defensive.

Keith: How did it affect you?

Fiona: I don't like conflict really, so I could feel my anxiety rising.

Keith: Were you involved in the discussions?

Fiona: Yes. I am there to present the figures. I felt a bit like a mediator. My job is to report the figures and offer advice, but they both wanted to use the figures for their own ends. I found myself trying to keep the peace, but also being misinterpreted.

Keith: Is that your role, keeping the peace?

245

Fiona: Not really. My role is to take care of the accounts and ensure the company finances are reported accurately. I found the whole thing quite aggressive.

Keith: How did it impact your contributions to the meeting?

Fiona: I don't think I did contribute much, really. Partly trying to get a word in edgeways. And also holding back – I wanted to focus on one area but found that I couldn't get the words out.

Keith: How's it leaving you now, as you're talking about it?

Fiona: A bit anxious. And frustrated – frustrated with them and frustrated with myself. Angry, if I'm honest. Tense. And feeling I might be letting them down and myself down too. I'm meant to be active in these meetings.

Keith: I'm wondering where you might be holding that tension. Are you noticing anything in your body now?

Fiona: In my chest.

Keith: In what way?

Fiona: It's feeling tight. From my chest up to my throat. [Pointing to the area].

Keith: What's that like to get your words out?

Fiona: It's difficult. It feels like there's something stuck there and I can't get the words to my throat.

Keith: You told me in a previous session that you like to practice yoga.

Fiona: That's correct, I do.

Keith: What's one of the primary things they teach in yoga?

Fiona: Breathing.

Keith: Yes, just taking yoga breaths. Have you applied it in the meetings?

Fiona: No, I'd never thought of that.

Keith: Let's give it a go now. Just sit and notice it a minute. Just take a few deep breaths. Allow yourself to breathe in and out a few times, *taking full yoga breaths. [Pause for one minute.] What are you noticing, now you have been with it for a minute?*

Fiona: It's easing, calming. I'm not so tense now.

Keith: How are you feeling?

Fiona: More relaxed, calmer. I can breathe easier now.

Keith: I'd like to return to something you said earlier.

Fiona: OK.

Keith: You said, "My role is to take care of the accounts." What do you think of that phrase – taking care?

Fiona: It's how I feel, but now hearing you say it back to me, I'm not sure it's quite right. Maybe "manage the accounts" is better. Yes, that works well.

This vignette shows what can happen in a pressured situation when the individual – in this instance Fiona – has susceptibilities:

Head: Rationally and logically, she was attending a meeting because of her knowledge and expertise. She is highly professional and has the trust of the board to be appointed finance director. She is highly capable and professional.

Feelings: Emotionally, Fiona was feeling nervous about the meeting but was put more at ease at the start. Her response to the conflict, however, increased her emotions of anxiety, frustration and anger – and her desire to keep the peace.

Felt sense: The situation triggered a bodily reaction. The tightening in the chest, narrowing of the airwaves made her breathing shallower and more difficult to speak, literally compressing her ability to contribute. The body's muscles cannot be tense and relaxed at the same time. Muscles don't work that way. (Imagine the athlete whose muscles are tense as she lines up for the Olympic 100 metres final. No athlete can perform at their best with tense muscles. At best, they will reach the finish line, at worst, they will pull a muscle.)

And it was a similar situation for Fiona, lining up for her equivalent 100 metres. It was only by accessing her felt sense that she was able to become more aware of its grip on her in this context. By becoming aware of it, and just noticing it, this enabled her to become more in touch with herself, and thereby start to loosen its grip in the coaching room. She strengthened her connections with herself. She was better able to control her muscles – when to relax, when to tense them.

Rationally she knew what to do; emotionally she became agitated, and physically she put herself into a type of lockdown. Learning to accept the felt sense – and what is held within the body – might be the key for her to unlock the door. Notice how she then reconsidered her role with accounts from "taking care" to "managing".

Consider Fiona's experience in the context of these words from Richard Strozzi-Heckler, who writes that: "When we move our attention from the feeling self to the thinking self, we lose contact with much of life."

Those are strong words. By shifting her attention from her thoughts to the felt sense within her, Fiona became more grounded, more aware – and more capable of taking an active part in the meeting, rather than reacting to the emotional undercurrent in the room. Gendlin invites you to trust in your body, writing that: "Once your body is allowed to be itself, uncramped, it has the wisdom to deal with your problems." In this space, you will be dealing with such inner tensions with a "relaxed, loose body" – and definitely not an armoured body.

Accessing and integrating your felt sense

Imagine, for a moment, a lily on the surface of a pond. Its leaves lie flat on the calm surface of the water while the flower grows a short distance upwards and opens up towards the warmth and glow of the sun.

Allow yourself to appreciate the beauty of the flower rising atop the stem into the daylight. Imagine that as Fiona in full bloom. Confident, seen, appreciated, contributing, self-confident. Taking her richly deserved place with her colleagues. Seen and heard in meetings. Conveying her points both calmly and professionally.

Now drop below the surface of the water to the earth at the bottom of the pond.

The lily is able to flower – and occupy its rightful place in the pond – because of its secure roots. A solid base. Imagine that is Fiona's body – that is where her felt sense is located. But imagine if those roots are weak, or there is less opportunity to grow. The foundations are less; it feels less secure and might not flower so beautifully.

Lastly, think of the stalk – the communication passage between the blooming flower and the roots. All those messages flowing back and forth. All the nutrients drawn from the roots that enable the lily to reach to – and beyond – the surface and take its rightful place there with the other lilies. For a person, all the impulses and messages going backwards and forwards between the mind (the blooming flower), the body (the roots) via the stalk (the nerves and muscular connections). And imagine what happens if the stalk is compressed or stretched or injured. Communications will be impeded. So, if we consider the body-mind connection, think of it in terms of a strong felt sense throughout the body; a strong communication system that connects the body and mind together, holistically. These will allow Fiona to contribute more effectively in meetings.

Remember Fiona's breathing exercise. Inhaling the oxygen from the atmosphere, allowing it to enter her whole body. At its best, a seamless two-way process between body and mind; and mind and body.

Raising your awareness of your felt sense comes through noticing. And allow yourself just to notice. Don't analyse, don't interpret, don't allow your rational head to take over – just notice your felt sense.

Just notice.

The more you notice, the more you become aware. Simply attend to your body.

Many people alienate parts of their body. That doesn't help – it simply separates. A consequence of trauma is that of dissociation – separating parts of oneself. The journey back can be to integrate, to join together. To remember who we were before the traumatic episode(s). Think of the word remember – it is re-member, to bring things back together.

If you think of the lily metaphor, notice the connections. See yourself as an integrated, interconnected whole. See yourself holistically. All the parts are connected.

As you learn to attend to your body, simply notice. Where do you hold your tension? What little aches and pains pop up and where?

And notice the relaxation. Allow yourself to relax.

Notice your felt sense right now as you relax. Become aware of how your feet feel when standing or resting on the ground. Notice the feelings of sitting – and feeling supported – when you are relaxing in a chair. When lying in bed, allow yourself to feel your whole body against the sheets on the mattress.

Exercise

First, allow yourself to relax and think of three events that lead to a reaction in you:

- One that leads to something you look forward to.
- One that leads you towards feeling relaxed.
- One that leads to tension and anxiety within you.

Complete the tables below in turn. You might want to give yourself a break between each.

Note: I am avoiding words such as 'positive' and 'negative' because I am inviting you just to notice. Let go of judgemental language.

Event	Felt sense What you notice in your body
Something you are looking forward to	

Event	Felt sense What you notice in your body
Something that generates a sense of relaxation	

Event	Felt sense What you notice in your body
Something that leads to tension	

When you have completed this exercise, use the space below to note down the effects this had on your felt sense:

CHAPTER 40

Think, feel, intuit, do

Just because you are using your intuition, it doesn't mean you are ignoring logic.

Here's a way of addressing issues. Allow yourself to consider a topic from three perspectives: head, heart, gut.

- What does your head think to do?
- How does your heart feel about the issue?
- How are you intuiting? What are you sensing from your gut instinct?

One of the recurrent themes of the English lockdown during the pandemic were repeated government statements that they were "following scientific advice". That suggests a focus purely upon the rational, scientific, evidence-based aspects of handling the pandemic.

People who make decisions purely from a rational perspective are following the logical approach. While the decisions were being made by the government that were described as being scientifically based, the government's own Office for National Statistics conducted a survey that discovered that people in lockdown were more concerned with their mental health than their general health. Does that, I wonder, bring into play feeling-based evidence? How those people felt about lockdown? And perhaps this can be extended to sensations within their gut instincts.

People who make feelings-based decisions are sometimes described as letting their hearts rule their heads. They are characterised as passionate people. Often it stops there. But what does your gut instinct say as well? To what degree do you allow this into the mix?

One way of looking at a decision-making process is to accommodate all three. In the diagram below, it is presented as the classic Venn diagram format – three characteristics, each with equal weight.

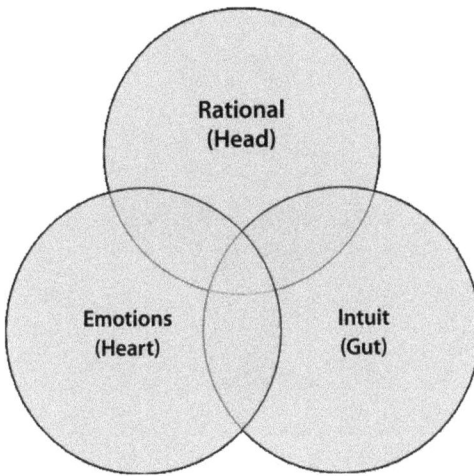

How do you make your decisions? Of course, this may vary from one context to the next. A professional/business decision might be characterised by greater rationality, while a personal/family decision might be dominated by emotions.

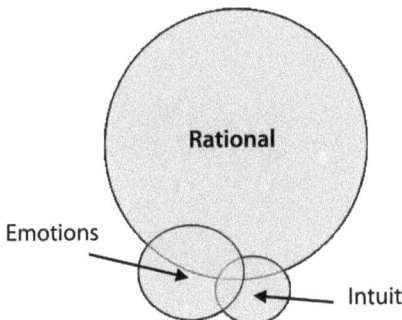

Look at the diagram above. In this instance, the decision is made mostly from a rational perspective, with emotions and intuition playing much smaller roles.

Below is another variation. A rational decision is made, with small input from emotions. Although emotions are available, they are largely bypassed. And intuition is ignored, bypassed or out-of-awareness.

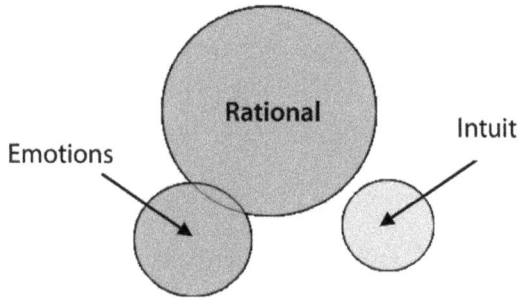

In this decision, intuition is dissociated from the decision-making or problem-solving process, and there is only a tenuous link between head and heart.

Grant Soosalu and Marvin Oka describe a three brains approach – that you can consider yourself as having three brains – one of which is located in the head, as you might expect, while the others are located in the heart and gut. And, according to the authors, each of these has separate functions.

This raises some interesting perspectives – and brings back the theme of emotional intelligence, explored in chapter 21. That approach focuses on thoughts and emotions – the head and the heart. Perhaps we can recall those occasions when our head says one thing, but our heart says another. And what does our gut, our intuition say? I recall a conversation with a friend, who was considering joining her parents' business. I asked her what her head thought about it. She described it as a sensible, safe decision. We then moved onto her heart – which was mixed. She loved her parents and wanted to help, but her feelings were also taking her in the direction of what she wanted to do – which was to forge her own career, to express her own identity. I then asked her what he gut might be saying. She paused for a moment, allowed herself to be open to her intuition and said, confidently, that her intuition was to develop her career away from the business. This would allow her to move back into the business at a future date, if she chose to. She was very content with her choice.

You might think about something as a good idea rationally, yet there is a sense in your gut that it's not quite right. It feels off. Imagine a conversation, for example, with a well-meaning friend. You are discussing a problem you have, and he comes up with a rational solution. It makes perfect sense. You might even agree with him – to some degree. Yet there is another part of you that hangs back, that doesn't feel quite right. You might have experienced this with other people – when it is oh-so-easy to make sense of their problem, and why-don't-they-just-do-what-you-advise-them-to-do?

Their behaviours or resistance might seem irrational, but seemingly irrational behaviours have rational explanations. Perhaps the word wisdom can be applied here. Wisdom, as distinct from knowledge. Perhaps wisdom brings in data from all three brains.

The authors contend that each of the brains has a 'highest' expression. For the head brain, it is creativity; for the heart brain, compassion; for the gut brain, courage.

Three words to bring together within you: creativity, compassion and courage.

Activity

Making decisions: the three circles approach

Allow yourself to consider a number of situations in which you set about solving problems and/or making decisions.

Think about different contexts, for example:

Context	Summary of the problem to be solved or decision to be made
At work	
With family	
Personal to you	
With friends	

Then, in the space below, use the decision-making circles approach to consider a typical decision to be made. Draw the three circles (gut, head, heart) in accordance with how influential each of these are in the different contexts. Make a note of any thoughts that come to mind when you consider each of them. Allow yourself to notice, without judgement.

At work	With family
Personal to you	With friends

When you have completed the exercise, reflect upon the following

What do you notice about your circles?

What experiences from your past might be influencing how you make decisions today?

How can you use your reflections in this chapter to guide your decision-making in the future? How might you 're-shape' your decision-making processes?

Chapter 41

Yoga: breathe, exhale and inhabit your body

Psychological stresses end up in your body. They can inhibit the body's functioning. Now is the time to fully inhabit (and not inhibit) your body.

We can learn to inhabit our bodies more fully – and differently – through our breathing and yoga. I have learnt valuable lessons from yoga, just two of which are as follows.

- The first is breathing and learning to breathe richly and more fully.
- The second is to stretch the body in ways that help me and then to breathe full yoga breaths in these extended (but not forced) positions.

Firstly, a series of rich and deep inhales and exhales. Breathing in, really breathing in, holding breath and then exhaling gradually, emptying the body of air as far as comfortably possible and then repeating the process several times.

Think of times when you feel stressed. Allowing yourself to breathe this way can be a great aid. A long, full exhale can help release tension you might be holding.

James Nestor has written an entire book on breathing – it's called *Breath: The New Science of a Lost Art*. In the introduction, he points out that the law of averages indicates that you will take some 670 million breaths in your lifetime – around 25,000 times a day. Maybe because we do so much of it and automatically that we often just take it for granted. But at what cost? He argues that many of us have lost touch with this essential function. His view is this has significant consequences for us – but learning to breathe fully and richly can have transformative effects upon us.

Consider the body mind as a single entity: all part of yourself. It's all too easy to get wound up or feel tension in the 'head' but everything is contained within your body. Allowing anxiety and tension to release from your body is an effective way of letting go, of relaxing. Allow it to flood out of your body and through your body and/or your feet into the ground below. Let it go.

Consider, for a moment, the types of phrases you might use and how these might be reframed.

Phrases that are often used	How the phrase might be spoken to elicit a different message
"I'm a bit out of sorts."	"I'm OK with myself, even though I'm not 100%."
"I'm not my usual self today."	"I'm sitting with a different aspect of myself today. I'm connecting."
"I'm all over the place today."	"I'm right here, right now."

The statements on the left suggest some disconnection or unresolved themes. Using the language in the right-hand column suggests a more integrated body/mind.

Sometimes when you are 'in your head' it is all too easy to forget your body. Simple, deep breathing exercises like this can help you to connect, to be more at one with yourself within your body. Notice where you are feeling the tension. Remember, muscles cannot be tense and relaxed at the same time, so this approach can be used to ease the tension. Breathe deeply, remain grounded. Allow yourself to become more integrated. Feel whole.

Practising yoga allows you to extend this throughout your body. That simple process of taking up a particular position and then allowing yourself to breathe in that place can work wonders for the body. Imagine the opposite. Imagine you recently slightly over-extended yourself. The surrounding muscles have tensed up into a more fixed, rigid position to protect that part that 'tweaked'. The challenge then is that the muscles need to be encouraged to come out of 'lockdown' that the body has imposed. One way is to stretch the muscle and then allow yourself to breathe in and out in that particular extended position. So that you are breathing in that new, expanded place, which allows your body to stretch, become acquainted with your new normal and then inhabit that new normal.

And consider those traumatic memories that may be held within your body, within your felt sense. They may have built up over the years or resulted from a single experience. Stretching and breathing via yoga can become your way of inviting yourself to ease into a new bodily position, to shift your felt sense, to loosen old rigidities and tensions.

And a word of caution, which links to 'what you don't want' from others, explored earlier in the book. We explored the fact that it doesn't always really help to talk with someone who might simply want to fix you or solve your problems for you. Perhaps the same applies in yoga. If you go to a yoga session and tell the yoga facilitator that you want to work on a particular part of your body, then there is the risk of the 'fixing' approach being applied. Perhaps there is a way that allows you to loosen within that area of your body, contained within the context of a whole, holistic, intuitive approach. Integrate the mind within itself, the body within itself and the body and the mind together, holistically.

As you breathe in, you breathe into yourself, as you breathe out, you exhale, you let go, you relax, you become more still.

CHAPTER 42

Mindfulness, meditation and awareness

Getting in touch with your mind.

To understand mindfulness, let's consider our awareness in two ways – directed awareness and undirected awareness.

Directed awareness is, simply, where you direct your awareness. Imagine a racehorse with its blinkers on. It looks forward; its focus is directed towards the finishing post. Blinkers on a horse limit opportunity for its peripheral vision. Quite simply, directed awareness has a narrow focus.

Imagine you have parked your car and are running to the station to catch a train. You are late. You are focused on getting to the train station, perhaps sprinting past other people to stake your place in the queue. You might alarm them as you go by, but you don't really notice – or care. You are concentrating on that ticket desk. You might be cursing over the slow traffic or how you mislaid your phone before you dashed out of the house. You arrive at the queue for the tickets. You see the train is due in five minutes and there are three people ahead of you in the queue. You think you have sufficient time. Then you realise the people being served want to renew their season tickets, or need things explaining to them, or start chatting amicably with the ticket sellers. Your tension rises, you find yourself muttering under your breath…

Does this sound familiar? You are most definitely in the directed awareness zone! And maybe you have your train blinkers on so much that you are missing many other things around you.

Undirected awareness is more open. It is about being receptive to what is available in your environment – and to what might emerge. If in **directed** awareness you are looking through a telescope to see the surface of the moon, then in **undirected** awareness you look up to the stars above, allowing yourself to take in the whole of the night sky. Then you start to notice more.

Let's return to the train station for a moment. When your undirected awareness is given air, you might notice the solidity of the ground beneath your feet as you walk towards the ticket office. Or the feel of the chill wind. Perhaps the smell of the coffee as you walk past the coffee bar. Or you hear the clunk-clunk-clunk of the goods train as it pulls its weighty load through the station. You can experience yourself and what is going on around you as wholeness. You're not directing your awareness but are opening yourself to all that is going on around you.

Directing your awareness can distance you from everything that is 'out there' to what is running around inside your head – your internal commentary, your interpretation, your analysis. You have shifted your life from being open to what's around you to riding along train tracks inside your head. You are no longer fully 'present' in your environment. Let's explore the limiting nature of directed awareness.

Case study

Ralph's story

"One day I was walking through the marketplace of a large city, near where I live. I was making my way to see an important client. I was focused on the meeting and was mentally preparing myself. Suddenly I heard a voice to my right, somewhere behind me, saying, "Hello, Ralph." I stopped suddenly and turned round. I had walked right past a woman who had been approaching me in the opposite direction. I hadn't even seen her. It was a colleague who I hadn't seen for over a year. I was inside my head, was lost in my thoughts and hadn't noticed her. I was *embarrassed. She had been ill for a year, suffering and then recovering from breast cancer. I apologised. I was so much in my head that I had become oblivious to my environment."*

Being dominated by one's own thoughts can be seen many times every day. Anxious car drivers who see the traffic light is changing from red to amber to green but still go over the traffic crossing to save themselves 30 seconds but endanger others. Their focus is their journey, their needs, possibly with huge consequences.

Or the person at work who never says "good morning" to others because she is so focused on the computer monitor in front of her eyes. While she concentrates on her work, others feel ignored. Her relationship with colleagues risks being undermined.

Undirected awareness allows you to be more open with what emerges – and what is going on around you. You have greater contact with other people and your environment – you turn down the voice in your head and become more attuned to your senses.

Quite simply, you notice more. You live more. And you can turn that attention within too. The practice of mindfulness or meditation, where you sit or lie, encourages you to move to undirected awareness. To notice parts of your body as you allow yourself to observe. There are those moments when the mind can wander – and then gently return – and then you allow it to settle as you develop the skills to reflect in a more mindful manner.

In these moments, you can become more aware of the universe that is out there and are better able to integrate it with the universe that exists inside you.

To develop mindfulness skills, just notice. Allow yourself to become aware of your senses – see, feel, touch, hear, smell. Avoid judgement, analysis and interpretation. Allow yourself to be open to more undirected awareness.

Chapter 43

Who do you want to be?

Becoming who you want to be is true, deep transformation.

There's a description of coaching created by Eric Parsloe and Monika Wray which proposes that coaching can enable someone to "become the person they want to be". I love this description of the purpose of coaching. It offers up so many possibilities.

Yet it also has a challenge, which I will pose as a question. Do you yet know who that person is that you want to be? If your answer is 'yes', then great! But perhaps you are one of those people who haven't yet really given it much thought. Perhaps you can't answer that question just yet.

Now could be a good time to start.

It's helpful to distinguish between *who you want to be* and *what you might want to do*. And also to see how these might be connected.

Case study

Rebecca's story

Rebecca was an extremely successful sales manager. Married, she was the breadwinner in the family.

Her daily commute lasted 90 minutes each way to central London. When her first baby arrived, she worked as long as possible before the birth and then was back at her desk six weeks later. Two years later, baby number two arrived. In our first coaching session after her second child was born, she said to me, "I don't want to carry on working in London any more. I want to help my husband to run his business."

There was an element of both "being" and "doing" in her decision. The "being" was the main one, by a country mile. Foregoing the career to spend time with her family was the critical choice in her decision. Carrying out her husband's administration (bookings and finances) wasn't a full-time job. It was a lifestyle choice.

She was pretty clear on who she wanted to become.

Activity

Who do you want to become?

Who do you want to become? If that is different from who you are now?

You might wish to consider this in three steps:

1. Allow yourself to be in a comfortable place.
2. Think creatively: allow yourself time and space to explore what this person {you) may be like.
3. Reflect upon and absorb your learning from this activity.

Let's look at the three steps in turn.

Get yourself comfortable

Allow yourself to be in a place that is conducive to your relaxed, free thinking. This might be a particularly comfortable chair at home, for example. Or perhaps your meditative moments emerge over a steaming cup of coffee in a café, surrounded by the hum of other customers. Or sitting in your garden. Or walking through the beautiful countryside. Whatever works best for you. And think of the time of day, too, when you will be relaxed.

When and where I feel relaxed

Get creative

A powerful technique is to visualise the future. What might it look like? You don't have to visualise just with your eyes though. What does it feel like? Or what might you be hearing in the future? You might want to visualise a year or several years ahead. Perhaps five or 10 years. Or even 20 years. Allow yourself to be open to possibilities.

You might want simply to reflect upon this, or you might want to put things down on screen or on paper.

The simple act of treating yourself to a sketchpad or notebook can be a good start:

- A sketchbook with a set of coloured crayons or coloured pens. You could draw what this might be like.
- A notebook can be the start of a reflective journal for you as you write down your thoughts.

Or you might want to pick up nearby objects and put them into shapes and patterns on a table or on the floor to envisage your possible future.

Allow yourself to be free of judgement here. Just write down or sketch whatever emerges.

The person I want to become

Reflect and notice

Next, just notice what you have created – either your words and/or sketches or shapes or whatever medium you have chosen.

- Notice what you have created.
- What emerges for you as being significant?
- How does the future relate to how you are today?

Again, do so without judgement. Allow yourself to be open to possibility.

Reflections

Summary

Answer the two questions below.

From this exercise, what stands out the most for you in your imagination for your future?

What one thing will you do to move towards that vision? To start connecting the vision with where you are now?

CHAPTER 44

Ask yourself the miracle question

"Miracles are not contrary to nature but only contrary to what we know about nature." St. Augustine.

Sometimes in life, it seems that you can't find a solution. Everything feels hemmed in. It's as if you're in a deep forest and are struggling to find a path to get out. Or it's as if you have tried everything, and you just keep coming back to where you started. One door has slammed shut, and then so does the next one.

If that's the case – or even if not – then here's a technique you might like to try. And it just involves you asking yourself a question. And then, of course, doing some thinking and answering it. It's called the miracle question. The miracle question can be found in solution-based therapy.

It is based upon a question that invites you to set yourself a goal. Linda Metcalf has written a whole book based upon the miracle question. Imagine you are asleep tonight and, while you sleep, a miracle happens. Then, when you wake the next day, the miracle has happened – a miracle in your life. What might that be? She invites you to consider what you will see yourself doing, thinking or believing.

That's the question you can ask yourself.

Activity

The miracle question

Apply the miracle question to yourself and write down the answer. As you then reflect upon this:

- What do you notice?
- How might that make a difference for you?
- How could you be, or what could you do that would take you closer to that miracle?

What is the answer to your miracle question?
What do you notice?
How might that make a difference for you?
How could you be, or what could you do, that would take you closer to that miracle?

Chapter 45

Water for wellness

It's difficult to underestimate the depth, intimacy and benefits of our relationships with water.

Your first home was in the embracing and nurturing waters of your mother's womb, so it's no surprise that we often have a deep relationship with water – even if, perhaps, we don't consciously think about it. In Western countries, we have become so accustomed to water pouring from a tap that we take it for granted. We don't generally have that problem of turning on the tap and never being sure if water will flow or not. And we don't have to walk to the nearest well to get water. It's easy to take water for granted – but, like the air we breathe, our lives depend upon it.

Water is so versatile. It will fill any empty shape. It can become as solid as hard ice or fall as snow or hail. It can steam. It can be still or carbonated or gently (or strongly) flavoured. On a water products website, I discovered no less than 55 different brands of water, offering almost 200 different water drinks.

Water provides us with a host of opportunities to help on a healing journey to wellness. It allows us so many sensory experiences:

- Taste and feel of an iced drink of water.
- Smell of rain in the air.
- Cooling drops of rain on your head and body on a hot summer's day.
- Sound of raindrops bouncing off a roof.
- Feel of seawater spray exploding over rocks.
- Sight of dramatic clouds heralding a storm.

- Tingling chill (or warmth) of stepping into the sea.
- Vista of a majestic ocean at sunset.

Water allows life to grow – and that includes your life too. There are so many ways you can use water as a resource to help you on a healing and developmental journey.

Shower

The simple act of having a hot shower allows you to experience the relaxation of a jet of hot water flowing over you. Imagine you have had a long day at work, and you are carrying a lot of stress in your shoulders. Allow the shower to flow across the shoulders for 10 minutes or more. If you can, then adjust the showerhead to focus the water, or if you can pulse the water, then that can help. Or have a gentler rain shower. Or if it's a hot day, then perhaps the cooling waters will feel reviving and refreshing.

Elsewhere in this book, we considered the exploration of your body to see where tension might be held. You might wish to allow the warming water to soak into this area of your body; to give it some tenderness to counter the tightness. This is particularly effective with pulsed showers.

A hot bath

Such an old remedy! The relaxing and cleansing luxury of a hot bath at the end of the day, shortly before you go to bed to maximise the healing benefit. Enough said.

A long, cold drink

Allow yourself to savour the simple joy of a glass of water. No E numbers, no sugars, no additives, just water. Infuse it with a slice of fruit. Warm water can be so comforting. Drunk widely in Asian countries (and often provided with meals at restaurants) it is so distinct from cold water. It can also be very relaxing last thing at night. It is a lovely way to care for your inner self.

Go for a swim

If you are able to, then go for a swim. Allow yourself to be held by the water. If you are comfortable, then allow yourself to immerse yourself fully and swim below the surface too.

If you can't swim, then there is no time like the present. If you join a beginners' lesson, then expect there will be other people in the same position as you. You won't be alone with your concerns. A great goal is to be able to be in the water comfortably without your feet touching the bottom of the pool. It will work wonders for your confidence, both in and out of the water.

Swimming in the sea – give yourself the opportunity, if possible, to enjoy a swim in the sea. Feel the softness of the sand beneath your feet. Or safely try river or lake swimming.

Appreciate the sea

There's something special about sitting on a beach to watch the sun sink slowly over the horizon. That magical time when the light fades, the heat of the day has passed, but it is not yet dark. And when darkness has fallen, just notice how much more your hearing becomes attuned to the hypnotic, rhythmical sound of the sea as the waves break onto the beach and then recede again.

And take a walk along the beach first thing in the morning, before it becomes busy. The air is clearer at this time of day.

Walk along a river or lake

Take a stroll along a riverbank or along the shore of a lake. See the wildlife, embrace the natural environment, watch the reflections.

Allow yourself to feel grounded in nature. If you live in a city, relax into the cityscapes alongside the river or canal banks.

Make the most of the rain

Allow yourself to get wet! The first signs of rain see many people grabbing coats and putting up umbrellas. Sometimes you know you're just going to get wet. Make the most of it!

For many people, water is in plentiful supply. Many of the suggestions above are simple, straightforward and free to do. You don't need to do much to enjoy a plentiful reward. Perhaps we can all heed the words written by Jane Austen: *"Where the waters do agree, it is quite wonderful the relief they give."*

Lastly, we cannot conclude without mentioning the ironing. A necessary chore for many but a relaxing, meditative activity for others. Fill the iron with water, let it boil, and it becomes steam (or spray) which allows us to iron the creases out of our clothes. And just think how that metaphor works for us too – whether the water is hot, warm, cool, or cold – its different qualities can be used to help us iron out some of the creases in our inner selves.

Chapter 46

Connecting with your environment

Why it's good to ground yourself in your garden.

Our natural environment provides us with many opportunities for grounding and allowing ourselves to connect with the natural environment.

Indeed, basic grounding can start with feeling real contact with the earth.

Plant both feet firmly on the ground and allow yourself to connect with planet earth. Earth, after all, is everyone's home. Ultimately, we have no other home. There is no planet B, so let's all treat our global home respectfully.

One of the most meditative and grounding pastimes you can undertake is gardening – and you don't even need a garden for it!

At any moment in time, you can have your feet firmly planted on the ground, engage your senses with the particular plant that you are holding and, by using both hands, use both sides of your brain. It becomes very absorbing and allows you to get into the zone of gardening.

If you have a garden, you have ample opportunities not only to 'do' the activity but also to allow yourself to 'be' in the moment.

Perhaps you only have a small garden or a back yard that is concreted over. Simple, get potting. Or perhaps you don't have any outside environment – then bring the garden indoors, either into your home or on a balcony or window ledge if possible.

One of the benefits of lockdowns was people's connections with their gardens and with plants. Plants bring colour, shapes and variety – and fragrances that enrich the senses. And there was a boom in home-grown fruit and vegetables.

Creating and tending a natural environment in this way enables both connectivity and growth. You are connecting with life. And through connecting with the natural world, you are connecting with yourself.

Have you considered growing plants from seed? All you really need is soil, a windowsill, seed tray, a base to contain water – and, of course, the seeds!

Sue Stuart-Smith has written a lovely book called *The Well Gardened Mind: Rediscovering Nature in the Modern World*. She writes that "when we sow a seed, we plant a narrative of future possibility".

Lastly, growing plants will help climate change issues – you are also helping the environmental challenges that we face. So, there is not only an important renewal and regeneration agenda for you, but also for the environment.

And, perhaps, planting seeds in the ground is also a metaphor for you planting your seeds for your future. Then nurture them and watch what they can become!

Chapter 47

Miro's story: old traumas, new beginnings

I first met Miroslav Reljić nearly a decade ago in a virtual learning environment.

Miro had signed up for an online coaching programme that I was delivering at the time. It introduced delegates to life coaching and was designed to give them a 'taster' of the topic.

An important part of the course was a coaching demonstration session, in which I would coach one of the delegates in front of the group.

Miro volunteered to be my 'client' for the 30-minute session. It takes a lot of courage for a delegate to put himself forward – and courage was one of the first things I noticed about him. His chosen topic was whether to progress a career in coaching or not. I remember this being a positive session.

It must have been because the following autumn, Miro turned up for a coach training programme that I was delivering at the Institute of Continuing Education at the University of Cambridge. He completed the Diploma qualification with ease.

Throughout the programme, I was struck by Miro's humour, energy and enthusiasm. He has a great way of combining profound topics with a lightness and an energy that suffuses his whole being and lights up a room.

Miro has gone on to become a highly successful coach and author.

His story, starting on the next page, is powerful and triumphant. It shows levels of resilience that have enabled him to deal with the trauma of growing up in a wartime environment, becoming a refugee and building a new life, many thousands of miles away.

Here's his story…

Old traumas, new beginnings

When the NATO bombing of Serbia stopped on 10 June 1999, I received the visa to emigrate to Canada. Let me share my story with you.

Prior to this date, Belgrade was bombed for 78 days, and I was in my last year and last semester at the University of Belgrade, majoring in economics. Having lived through the civil war in Croatia, I already had five years of extensive shelling experience "under my belt". I knew that I had to organize my life despite the daily attacks from the air. Several years earlier, my father had told me:

> *"If you hear the sound of 'it' [the grenade], you are safe, but if you do not hear it, you are in trouble, and seek shelter at once."*

This was my mantra. I tried to live my life as if the war was not happening.

However, when I reflect on it now, I was emotionally numb. I was in denial and always on edge. I spent most of my time studying and trying to detach myself from the situation that was beyond my control. Studying calmed my anxiety. The university library was the place where I spent most of my time, as it made me feel safe. That's how I coped with the stress and trauma as a teenager, and I used the same strategy as a university student. I escaped the reality by creating my own bubble.

When the civil war in Croatia ended in September of 1995, I was sent as a refugee by the Serbian government to Pristina, Kosovo. In Pristina, I had decided that I would leave the Balkans for good.

I started mailing applications once a week to the Canadian Embassy in Belgrade, explaining the reasons why I wanted to emigrate to Canada. When I later moved to Belgrade in 1997, I continued with sending applications. Between 1995 and 1999, I believe I wrote around 200 application letters.

For years I didn't get any response back, and most of my friends thought that I was wasting my time. I had doubts myself. However, I continued writing as I could reflect and grieve my losses.

In late March 1999, I received the first positive response from the embassy, and the Canadian immigration process from then on was fast. I passed all the interviews. I knew that I would have to make a quick decision regarding my studies and that if I were to leave Serbia, I would not be able to finish my degree. Also, as the recipient of the National Railway Scholarship, I had a guaranteed job offer upon completing the studies. So that opportunity would have been lost as well. My parents were against my emigration. However, I'd had enough of wars, and the decision was to leave Serbia the moment I got the visa.

When I received the confirmation letter that my immigration papers were approved, I was over the moon. I still remember the departure time and date: noon on 13 June 1999. The embassy didn't give me a lot of time, but I was mentally prepared. Because the war had ended three days earlier, there was no air traffic between the capital of Serbia and other European cities. The only way to leave the country was to bus it from Belgrade to Budapest.

The United Nations High Commissioner for Refugees (UNHCR) office had chartered the bus. My travel itinerary was as follows: at noon, meet with the group in front of the museum of Nikola Tesla. Board the bus and travel to Budapest. From there, we would fly to Paris, France and the next day, on 14 June, we would fly to Montréal, Canada. In Montréal I would catch a flight to my final destination, Calgary. In total, 50 hours of travel that in regular circumstances would take about 20 hours or less.

I boarded at noon, and I sat next to the window seat all the way at the back of the bus. The bus filled up quickly with about 25 people on it. Most of the passengers were couples in their late 20s and early 30s. I remember it was a beautiful sunny day. However, inside the bus, the atmosphere was glum. No one was smiling. Just a lot of worrying and uncertainty about the trip. What if we get turned around at the Serbian border? What if we get turned around at the Hungarian border? There were a lot of "what ifs".

As refugees, we were stateless and didn't belong to any country. We travelled on UNHCR travel certificates.

At half past noon, a UNHCR officer entered the bus to make sure that our paperwork was correct. She was efficient and firm. One couple didn't have their Serbian exit visa stamped and signed. "I am sorry, but you will not be able to travel today," the officer said. She continued: "You will have to leave the bus and sort this out." It was the husband who didn't have his documents properly filled, and the wife said: "You never listen to me. I knew this was going to happen. It is your fault!" While the family drama was unfolding, I drifted away, trying to catch a glimpse of my parents. They were outside and waving goodbye.

I waved back. I put on my brave face and I smiled. On the inside I had mixed emotions of both sadness and excitement. I was sad as I knew that I would not be able to see them for many years.

However, I was excited about Canada! Although it was thousands of kilometers away from the Balkans, I needed the physical distance and space. I was on the bus! I had done it!

We left Belgrade at one o'clock in the afternoon, and we didn't have any problems at the border. We arrived in Budapest around midnight. Our group was booked at a hotel near the airport. The moment we arrived at the hotel, I knew that we would not be able to sleep as there was a party on the main floor. This was not a regular party as there were strippers and loud music.

The situation was surreal. Less than 12 hours before, we lived in a country that was at war and isolated from the rest of the world. I joked with my fellow travelers: "OK, people, let's not get carried away here as we still need to catch the plane in a few hours." One of the ladies from the group said to her husband: "Did you hear that? And by the way, you are married! I am watching you!" We all laughed. It was the first time that we laughed.

We left the hotel at 3am to catch the 5am flight to Paris. The one-hour flight was quick, and we landed at Charles de Gaulle, Paris, at 8am. Since we were all travelling to Canada, a few people who spoke English convinced the group to go to Terminal 1 and wait there for our Air Canada flight. Around 10am, I started questioning that something was not right. I was looking at the arrival and departure monitors and concluded that we need to go to Terminal 2. I made a decision to leave the group. Others followed shortly and we were all able to catch the flight.

When I landed in Montréal on June 14, I was so jet-lagged that I mistakenly boarded a connecting flight to Halifax instead of Calgary. I found my seat and I made myself comfortable. I remember looking outside the window, and I admired the beauty of a parked Air Canada airplane.

Minutes before the take-off, I asked a fellow passenger with a big smile: "Calgary?" and he replied with surprise: "No, Halifax!" I took my carry-on, and I ran as quickly as I could to catch the flight to Calgary. The Air Canada airplane that I had seen was the plane that I was supposed to be on. Both airplanes were leaving at the same time, but one was flying to Eastern and the other to Western Canada. I arrived in Calgary just before midnight. I was exhausted, but happy.

It was a new chapter in my life. I brought with me enthusiasm and a positive attitude, but I also carried my old traumas. However, I had an unrelenting resolve to keep moving forward and was looking forward to the new beginnings.

What was the worst thing about the bombings for you as a teenager?

An immense sense of loss. The loss that shook me to the core. I remember playing basketball with a friend one evening, and the next day he was dead. The bomb hit his car and the car went up in flames. I heard the news when I was on my way to school.

Even after 30 years, I can clearly remember that summer evening. I remember every single detail, the sound of a basketball bouncing off the asphalt, our jokes and laughs.

The following day, he perished in an instant. There was a sense that human life is worthless. That was the worst thing about the bombings. It was indiscriminate and dehumanizing.

What was the worst thing about leaving your homeland?

I think it was being uprooted. Since I was 16 years old until 22, I lived in four different countries, and I was always in transit. I missed my mother's homemade apple pie.

How would you describe the old traumas you were carrying with you?

Great question. I still carry them, and I have a lot of flashbacks. I would describe the old traumas as an annoying cousin who I do not want to be friends with. Because we are a family, I cannot cut him off, and he can show up unexpectedly and uninvited at my place at any time. The old traumas are like that. They pop up once in a while and remind me that they are still there. Over the years, I've learnt how to cope with them.

What was it like for you, starting your new life in Canada?

In Canada, I started from a clean slate. I really liked that. I was not dreading the new beginnings like many other immigrants that I met at the time, but instead I felt liberated to create a life I wanted. Starting from zero was an opportunity to learn and grow.

My sister, who moved to Calgary in 1996, helped me with the initial settlement. I spoke limited English. Being a "Chatty Cathy", I was frustrated because I couldn't express myself. That frustration motivated me to study even harder. I was adamant to learn English and go back to school and finish my economics studies.

I found a couple of survival jobs, including one cleaning offices in downtown Calgary. I remember cleaning one office on the 26th floor, and I told myself that within five years I will be working in a building like this.

I had a vision and clear goals. My prediction was almost spot-on. After graduating with a BA degree in economics in 2004 from the University of Calgary, I got my first professional job in 2005. For a dozen years, I worked as a business analyst, trainer and management consultant for oil and gas companies, before I turned to coaching for change full time in 2013.

Having a clear vision of what I wanted to achieve was really important. When one moves to a new country, a lot of people get sucked into their own communities and they become stuck. It feels safe and comfortable to stick with your "own" people. I remember an acquaintance trying to discourage me by saying: "You want to go back to school! Are you crazy? You are better off delivering pizza." There is nothing wrong with delivering pizza. I've done it.

However, I also had my goals and plans to achieve. In addition, as a gay man I didn't fit within my community. I had moments where I said to myself: "I didn't cross 10,000 kms to be ostracized by the people who speak my mother's tongue but are perfect strangers and are discriminating against me." This was not going to happen.

If I couldn't control my life when I was growing up, I certainly could when I moved to Canada. That decision helped me avoid trauma. I found new friends, and I built a new life in a wonderful country.

What I'm noticing about you moving forward includes having a clear vision, goals and plans; massive amount of drive, determination and resilience; not accepting other people's words and behaviours if not appropriate; choosing your friends; taking control. Was there anything else that really helped you at that time – or now?

When I make a decision, I stick to it. I will hear other people's opinions; however, I will take them with a grain of salt. I know my capabilities, and I know my strengths and weaknesses. When my friends tried to dissuade me from pursuing full-time English and economics studies, although they had valid concerns, deep down I knew that I could do it, and I did it.

Trusting myself and not second-guessing my decisions has helped me in the past and is helping me now.

One of the things I have noticed about you is a tremendous amount of optimism. How has this helped?

Optimism is like a magic wand that one can use to overcome challenges and ward off the naysayers. Being an optimist has helped a lot as I can "see" opportunities where other people cannot see them yet, or they fear too much of "what ifs" and unknowns.

A positive outlook on life, no matter what comes your way, has to be nurtured, so that in a tough situation you can take the magic wand and say, "I am going to be OK. Tomorrow is another day." When I say this out loud, I believe in this statement 100 per cent.

I remember when you were exploring coaching and attended an introductory online coaching course that I was facilitating. You volunteered to be the 'client' in a coaching demonstration session in front of the other students, and the topic you chose to be coached upon was whether you wanted to become a professional coach. What impact did that 30-minute online coaching session have for you?

That 30-minute online coaching session had cemented my decision to pursue coaching as a profession. After the session, I said to myself: "I want Keith to be my tutor and I want to learn from him." Shortly after, I applied for the Diploma in Coaching programme at Cambridge University.

Even six years later, I still remember the first session. It had a lot of flow, and the questions you asked helped me mobilize my energy. I am very grateful for that because after graduating from the programme, I started a successful coaching practice focusing on resilience and change. In addition, since my graduation, I've authored two books, and I would not be able to do it if I didn't have an increased awareness of what I offer.

What suggestions would you give to someone reading this book who might be going through a tough time?

I would say that please find the time to acknowledge the tough times that you are going through. It may not be intuitive, and it may hurt, but I think it is really important to acknowledge the situation you are in.

For example, when I became a refugee, I said: "I just lost everything." First time when I lost a job in Canada, I said: "I lost a job."

This is an important step that is often overlooked, and it helps with grieving and acknowledging the loss.

Second, in your journey you are not alone. Please try to reach out to people who have experienced similar difficulties/traumas in their lives.

As humans we spend a lot of time in our "heads" thinking and rethinking different "if" scenarios. What "if" this didn't happen, or what "if" I was not there. This inner monologue can go on and on. What "ifs" are draining and not helpful.

When we speak with people who have experienced similar difficulties, then there is a mutual understanding. Try to join a support group. If that is not possible, then maybe you create one. I didn't have a support group in Canada, so I created my own Facebook community that now has more than 2,000 members. It is important to reach out and talk.

Try not to bottle up your emotions and feelings as that can lead to depression, low-self-esteem and it can cause many health issues. In summary, to successfully go through tough times, I believe that it is important to acknowledge the loss and then talk about it with others who have experienced similar trauma/loss.

Miro, you write that: "The old traumas are like that. They pop up once in a while and remind me that they are still there. Over the years, I've learnt how to cope with them." How have you learnt to cope with them?

There are two coping mechanism that I use on a daily basis: asking questions and practicing self-compassion.

Asking questions – first, rather than suppressing my feelings, I've learnt to "communicate" with my traumas in order to reassure myself that I am all right. The key for me is to ask questions. For example, "How am I feeling when I am having a flashback?" or "How is my energy today?" and/or "Where is it in my body?" If I am feeling down, I will say, "I am feeling sad and that is OK. I am going to be OK." I have this inner dialogue for as long as I need it to feel reassured. Sometimes it lasts a minute and sometimes goes on for half an hour or longer.

Second coping mechanism is practicing self-compassion. For example, if I notice cramps in my stomach as a result of anxiety, I will put the hand over the stomach, and I say: "I love my tummy. Everything is OK." I believe that frequently "communicating" with my traumas has helped me lift the emotional weight off my shoulders – and has enabled me to successfully move forward.

You also write about a vision, goals and being in control of your life. What have been the most significant things that you have done – or how have you been – that have allowed you to build the life that is right for you?

I've been blessed to live in Canada. Canada has provided me with security that I needed in order for me to grow and express my creativity. Through my pro-bono workshops, I've coached thousands of newcomers on resilience and change. For that work, I was awarded the Royal Bank of Canada Top 25 Canadian Immigrants Award in 2017 and the Immigrant of Distinction Award for Community Service in 2018. I am proud to be the only Canadian who was selected three times in a row to coach executive MBA students at the UK's prestigious Cambridge Judge Business School, 2016, 2017 and 2018 cohorts.

Parallel to this, I was working on two book projects that were published in 2019. The first was a coaching book that I've co-authored with my colleagues Karen Root and Julian Brunt, who live in the UK and whom I met through the Diploma in Coaching programme at Cambridge. The book is titled *Insights into effective coaching: an interactive guide for helping you to find the right coach and getting the best results from your coaching.* The second book is a language and culture book titled: *The people of Bukovitza: authentic words, poems, stories and traditions of the Serbian people of Bukovitza and Dalmatia.* This book was my attempt to preserve the language and culture of the Serbian people from Croatia that has been lost due to the civil war.

What advice would you give to someone who has also experienced trauma and is seeking to move forward with their life?

Please try to find the courage to forgive yourself.

When you forgive yourself, you are back in control of your feelings and emotions. If you are traumatised it is highly likely that you were not in control of the situation, and of the individual(s) or the circumstances that had caused the trauma.

Please let me share how I do it:

First, I start with the hard stuff that will cause a lot of heavy emotions and an emotional release (usually through tears):

- I forgive myself. I forgive myself and acknowledge that the civil war was imposed upon me. I couldn't do anything; I was sucked into it. I am not a victim. (Notice a positive statement at the end.)
- I forgive myself. I forgive myself that I couldn't say a proper goodbye to some dear friends who died during the war. I am sorry that I didn't as it was out of my control. I still think of you every day and I love you.
- I forgive myself. I forgive myself that I was bullied as a gay teen for five years prior to and during the civil war. I couldn't influence other people's hatred or control it. I followed my own path and for that I am grateful and proud.

Second, I focus on lighter emotions/statements:

- I forgive myself. I forgive myself that I am a human with all my fears and hopes. Life is good!
- I forgive myself. I forgive myself that Covid-19 has caused a lot of upheaval in my life. I will bounce back.
- I forgive myself. Of course, I do. I am in control of my life.

It is a powerful exercise. Feel free to try it if you want. It works for me.

Activity

Miro's forgiveness model.

Using the table below, complete the sentences. Complete the first half (the topic) and then follow this with a positive statement. We have left spaces for three of these but add more if it helps you.

I forgive myself. I forgive myself ....

Then followed by a positive statement ....

PART 8

Awareness into action: stepping up your trauma recovery journey

In this section, we explore opportunities for you to empower yourself and to connect – both with others and with yourself. Its emphasis is to build your personal awareness, release your energy and then to engage in activities that will create movement within you. We conclude by suggesting a range of activities that you can undertake on your healing journey towards integration and connectivity.

Allowing yourself to be fully present wherever and whenever you are in your life is a fundamental building block on this journey. We start with this concept and then move on to consider some fundamental changes that can be easily introduced to move forward on the trauma recovery journey.

Let's not delay!

CHAPTER 48

Being in the present

Life can only be lived in the here and now.

The here-and-now is the present moment. The present moment is our existence right here, right now. It is the place where our power lies.

- The here and now is what is happening now.
- It is awareness of what is.
- It is about being fully present in the moment.

It is what is. Not what might be or might not be. Not what could be or couldn't be. Not what should be or shouldn't be. Not what ought to be or ought not to be. Not daydreaming out of the window. Not churning over the past. Not lost somewhere. Not living in the past or perpetually worrying about the future.

Life is about being fully present now. Here and now is what is happening in the present moment.

We can learn to become more present, aware in each moment, and aware as we move forward, moment to moment.

Part of the journey of overcoming trauma and memories of very difficult experiences is to be engaged in the present moment:

- To be in the moment.
- To live in the moment.
- To show up fully present.

- To dissolve any tendencies to dwell in the past, which limit your ability to access your power in the present moment.
- To learn to have your 'home screen' set to your awareness in the present, not your history channel.

For example, if you are locked in the past, with continuous flashbacks, repetitive patterns or a subconscious 'grip' on your reality, then it will inhibit your ability to fully show up in the present moment.

This unfinished business from the past leaves residual tensions which interfere with your ability to be present in the here and now. Even worse, unfinished business from a traumatic experience can leave you stuck. This is a journey of loosening the tight grip that those unpleasant experiences might hold on you. Thereby tying up your energy. Letting go of the past – dealing with the unfinished business – will release more of your energy. At the same time, it's integrating thoughts and feelings, mind and body. From dissociation to integration.

Then you can experience life at a richer level and go on to envision and create greater possibilities for yourself.

Remaining aware

Too often in life, it's all too easy to let ourselves be taken over by what's going on inside our heads. Take this awareness with you as you go through your life – in each situation you encounter.

Perhaps you are walking through some woods or riding a bicycle through the city. Or cooking a meal or taking a train journey. Allow your awareness to just be.

Turn down your head chatter, and literally allow yourself to come to your senses. Be in the moment. Walking barefoot is a great way to become more aware of the earth below your feet, to ground yourself in awareness. To walk through your home and feel the cool tiles or the thick carpet beneath your feet.

Read through the example below and then read the subsequent suggestion I was given.

Just consider the man in his car, stuck in a traffic jam on the motorway. He says, "I wish I was out on the golf course." Or the woman in the office, who says, "I'd much rather be walking along a beach." Neither of them is in the here and now. They are not present in the moment.

And the suggestion I was given was this:

If you want to know where you want to be in life, look where your feet are.

He's in his car on the way to a meeting to earn money so he can pay his golf membership fees. The woman's job allows her to have sufficient cash to go to the beach at weekends.

The minute that either of them would rather be playing golf or walking along the beach, then they will be. They are exercising choices. To earn money to be able to do those things.

I welcomed the advice I was given that day. It says a lot about empowerment, ownership and choices.

Chapter 49

Hear your words, change your language and shape your world for the better

You wouldn't pour acid on a plant and expect it to grow. Likewise, notice for any sharp or acidic words you might say to yourself. Look after yourself with nurturing and positive self-talk.

How often do we really pay attention to the language we are using? To what degree are we aware of the words we are using? On numerous occasions when I have been coaching people, I have made mental notes of their words and phrases. Then, when I have replayed their exact words to them, they have responded, with an air of disbelief: "Did I really say that?" Their own language has shocked them.

Imagine two people are in a busy road, laden down with shopping and hoping to hail a taxi. One person's self-talk is "I can always find a taxi", while the other person's mindset is "I am hopeless at finding a taxi". Who is the likeliest to discover a taxi first?

Our language is significant in influencing or reinforcing beliefs and behaviours. And we don't have to have experienced trauma to use words and phrases that don't do us any favours at all. Often, we switch off from our day-to-day use of words to our cost. Have you ever heard yourself saying any of the following?

Self-criticism

- "I've got no coordination…"
- "I can't paint…"

- "I'm no good at catching a ball…"
- "I'll never be as good as…"

The shoulds, musts and oughts

- "I must make sure that I…"
- "I really ought to…"
- "I need to cut the grass…"
- "I should have been a better mum…"
- "I'll try and go to the gym tonight."

Do any of these sound familiar? Here's a little experiment. Read the phrases above and notice what happens to your energy levels. [When writing them, my energy dropped somewhere through the floorboards.]

Words and phrases like the first four, which are often repeated on autopilot, might come from our belief systems. And then they reinforce those beliefs.

Were you born with those beliefs? I suggest not.

The end result of such beliefs is that you can end up going round in circles. When I am coaching clients, I might ask them to draw an image of how they are feeling or how they see a certain situation. More often than not, I am met with the same response. "I can't draw." Where did that belief system come from? When my children were very young – perhaps four or five years old – we would get the paints out, and within half an hour, pretty well most of the kitchen floor was covered in their paintings, laid out to dry. Roll on seven or eight years, and I suggest some painting and they told me they couldn't paint. How did that happen?

So as an adult, who says you can't paint? Or that you can't catch a ball? Or that you have no coordination? Repeated often, it becomes a belief system – something you believe to be true. And then imagine your interactions with other people. What sort of signal does this send out to other people? Have you paused to consider the possible consequences for you in your relationships with others? And how they will perceive you and respond to you?

The second set of statements lack conviction and energy. These are often the words of the child to appease or please the parent. When I hear them, I sense there will be inaction rather than action, coupled with emotional and physiological consequences, such as guilt and a sense of heaviness.

Consider two distinct but interrelated factors:

- General critical self-talk.
- The specific words you use.

Critical self-talk becomes a self-fulfilling prophecy. An example of this is:

"Why does it all go wrong for me?"

The individual who says this has become very alert to some kind of mishap, however slight. It has become very figural. There is a rigid mindset. Does it really always go wrong? Or perhaps it is perceived as a disaster because things didn't turn out perfectly. Something not working to perfection can easily fuel the fire of this irrational self-belief.

And notice how the critical self-talk plays out in specific words:

- "I am weak because I didn't stand up to him…"
- "I feel such a victim…"
- "I should have been stronger…"
- "I let the children down by not…"

Phrases such as these are like chains around the body. Except you can't 'see' these chains and have become numb to the weight of them.

As suggested previously, read the words out loud and notice what happens to your energy. It can feel like a dead weight compressed on your chest – and that might be what you are dragging along with you in life. So, it's time to cut loose the chains. And a simple way is to use different words. If this applies to you, then I invite you to reframe your language and start to challenge your assumptions and beliefs. (And if you have noticed an energy drop, then put this book down and walk around the room, or make yourself a drink, to create movement and shift your energy. This will also illustrate how you can shift your energy levels.)

Please allow me to introduce a metaphor to illustrate the situation. Imagine you are a yacht on the ocean and are static – you are not moving at all. The reason you are static is that you have five anchors that have dropped to the bottom of the sea and are keeping you stuck. Cut the chains of the five anchors by eliminating the following five words from your vocabulary:

- Ought
- Need
- Must
- Should
- Try

And now think of some more constructive words.

Choose is a good word to use. "I choose to..." And let's remember the lovely phrase from Henry Ford. "If you think you can, you're right; if you think you can't, you're right."

- "I choose..."
- "I will..."
- "I am..."
- "I can..."
- "I do..."

You can also think about the language you might use if you have experienced trauma. What words do you use to describe the events and what has happened since? Do you consider yourself a trauma:

- Victim?
- Sufferer?
- Survivor?

Words such as these can be given unhelpful meanings.

In one sense a "victim" is someone who, for example, has been the victim of a crime. In a psychological sense, a "victim" can be interpreted as someone who is "weak". This puts a less helpful meaning upon the word.

Working as a professional coach, I didn't want to see myself as a victim. Paradoxically, however, acknowledging that I was a victim allowed me to move on. And no longer to perceive the word victim as a weakness, but as a tribute to my ability to survive, revive and thrive. I was a victim. I am no longer.

Similarly, describing yourself as a sufferer and/or survivor is a statement of fact, but it is also replete with meaning.

Consider also language such as "I procrastinate" or "I dither over decisions". Perhaps you are oscillating, considering different options. Perhaps you are not yet ready to make a decision.

And beware the human tendency to over-simplify matters and to describe people with labels:

"He is weak because he doesn't confront people…"

"She looked like a tart dressed like that. No wonder that…"

Such labels minimise and demean people and are really not helpful. Labelling others and self-labelling helps to keep people stuck in the midst of self-limiting beliefs and assumptions.

Do attend to your words and the meanings they convey. The activity below is designed to raise your awareness of your language and the impact it might have upon you.

Activity

Over the next few days, notice the language that you use as and when you talk about yourself, or those words that come to mind when engaged in tasks. There are three columns.

1. What are the words/phrases you hear yourself saying?
2. How could you re-word these?
3. What do you think and feel after you have used the new phrase?

I have provided some examples to help start the process and left the right-hand column for you to complete.

Tip: *when you are completing this exercise, pay attention to 'hot' words and phrases such as should, ought, need, must, try.*

Words and phrases you use	How could you re-state this?	What do you think and feel when you have used the new phrase?
It always goes wrong for me.	It didn't work out quite as I planned, but I can learn from that.	
I am weak because I didn't stand up to him.	I had the courage to leave him and haven't gone back.	

I should have left her earlier.	I left her when the time was right for me.	
I'm just a doormat when it comes to…	I can choose when and if to put other people first.	

How has this exercise left you thinking and feeling?

CHAPTER 50

Reaching and making decisions

Allow yourself to oscillate, allow yourself to mull things over.

For many people, making a decision can sometimes, perhaps frequently, feel difficult.

Allow me to make that more specific. Making the so-called 'right' decision. It's all too easy to slide into the position of sitting uncomfortably on the horns of a dilemma – between a 'right' decision and a 'wrong' decision. It can feel like you are:

- Between a rock and a hard place.
- Stuck between what you want to do and what you 'ought' to do.
- Wondering whether to take the high road or the low road.
- Leaping out of the frying pan and into the fire.
- Between the lesser of two evils.
- Damned if you do, damned if you don't.
- Stuck in the middle (with you).
- Pulled from pillar to post.

Somewhere, somehow, we can get stuck in making a decision. We criticise ourselves (and others label us too) for 'procrastinating'. And notice what happens to your energy levels when you are in this place. Becoming and being stuck in this place often feels restricting and limiting.

It is notable there are many well-known sayings for the decision dilemma. And notice the strength of the language. Clearly many people have experienced such dilemmas!

Firstly, it's important to consider how you think about decisions. Back in the 1980s, Peter Honey and Alan Mumford described us as having learning styles – and two of the learning styles they described are activists and reflectors. The activist acts first and thinks later. The reflector thinks first and acts later. The activist who works as a police car driver might want to reflect when involved in a high-speed car chase along a busy road. Alternatively, the reflector whose house is on fire might want to get a move on if he's wondering if he has time to save some valuables.

But what happens when we reflect and reflect, and we still can't see a way out? There are several ways that might assist our thinking.

1. **Faulty thinking: right and wrong decisions**
   It's too easy to get hooked on making a 'right' decision and the anxieties over making a 'wrong' decision. One way of looking at this is that you're not going to be making a wrong decision. You are making the decision that is right for you at the time, for whatever reason. This leads to (2), below.

2. **Go with the decision**
   Go with the decision and then, if you need to, amend your decision. When an airliner is flying through the air from London to San Francisco, it isn't actually flying to San Francisco a lot of the time. The winds are continuously buffeting the plane off its flight path – so it is continuously adjusting to keep on track. With jet stream winds recorded at well over 200mph, the journey can be quicker or slower. And when the plane hits turbulent air, the passengers all return to their seats and put their safety belts on. And the pilot continually makes adjustments along the way. These can be major decisions. If the conditions are bad, it sometimes might mean flying to a different airport or even turning back. And that can be fine too. We make decisions, adjust and amend decisions and so on.

3. **Trust in energy shifts**

   Once you reach a decision, you will shift your energy – and life will respond accordingly. Life will respond. But as well as external life and an external universe, there is an internal universe inside you too.

What happens when you make decisions?

As well as the universe 'out there', think about the universe inside you.

Consider your wonderful possibility, your infinite potential. Estimates vary, but it is suggested that the average human body contains well over 30 trillion cells. So, while you are oscillating over a decision, millions of your cells will be oscillating with you as you weigh up the options. And when you reach a decision, they will respond with you as you step into your new paradigm and become more of who you are.

Think about your skin – such an important contact point between the outside universe and your own 30+ trillion cells. There are 35 billion skin cells. That's no less than 35 billion opportunities for feeling and interacting with the world at large.

These are awesome statistics. So, when you feel stuck on making a decision, remember that you have a vast array of complexity working in harmony inside you all the time. Carl Zimmer writes:

"...the very fact that some 34 trillion cells can cooperate for decades, giving rise to a single human body instead of a chaotic war of selfish microbes, is amazing."

So, you are awesome and amazing! Please remember this.

Making decisions: give yourself three options

We looked earlier at the problem of being on the horns of a dilemma. Do you go this way or that way? Do you go for the rock or the hard place? The frying pan or the fire? Here's a good way of looking at a decision to be made. Give yourself three options.

It has been said that:

- If you only see one solution, you have a problem.
- If you see two options, you have a dilemma.
- If you have three ways out, you have a choice.

You may wish to consider more options as well. A dilemma can feel like a win or lose situation, so shifting it opens up new possibilities. To help broaden your perspectives – and perhaps think of new resolutions, you could ask yourself questions like these.

Ideally, think of a 'problem' you have that you think there might be only two ways out. Then ask yourself questions like these:

- What could you do?
- What else could you do?
- If you think of someone you respect, what would they suggest you do?
- If you were the boss of the company, what would you suggest?
- If you were president of your country, what would you suggest?
- If you were talking with someone who has the same problem as you, how would you advise them?

Activity

Exploring a problem: identify your options and weigh them up.

Step 1. Consider a decision that you are facing. Identify three options you could follow. Write them in the space below.

Step 2. When you have identified three options, complete the rows below to help you to reflect on your decision.

Step 3. Once you have completed the exercise, write down your reflections in the space below.

Questions to ask yourself	Write a summary of each option in the box below		
	Option 1	Option 2	Option 3
What does your head think about this?			
How does your heart feel about this?			
What would be the benefit for you?			
What would be the drawback for you?			
What would be the benefit for others?			

Questions to ask yourself	Write a summary of each option in the box below		
	Option 1	Option 2	Option 3
What would be the drawback for others?			
On a scale of 1-10, how committed are you to each of these?			
What's your intuition on this?			

Once you have completed the exercise, write down your reflections below.

Chapter 51

Build your support networks

Connect with yourself and connect with others.

Far too many people who have had traumatic experiences spend too long in states of loneliness and isolation. There can be an inclination to withdraw from others – but that only makes matters worse. Pulling away or isolating intensifies feelings of loneliness.

Yet even in groups, one can feel lonely. That strange sensation when you are with many other people yet feel curiously alone.

A good antidote is to build your own networks – plural. Traditionally, networks have been based around family, friends and work – but with the internet and social media, it is possible to network with others in ways that were unimaginable just a few years ago. Make and build contact with others.

Online: there is a lot of information out there. Not only can you research and develop your understanding of the effects of traumatic experiences, but trauma-focused websites also have discussion forums and links to groups. Online groups can feel both safe and risky. You can make remote connections with others, sometimes globally, who perhaps have had similar experiences. These forums do give you an opportunity to considerably reduce your isolation, even remotely. Indeed, the sense of safety through the virtual environment can also be beneficial.

Support groups: Support groups are helpful because of the benefits from shared experiences and shared understandings. Perhaps you move on from them but retain a few friendships. Being in groups where you are understood and accepted – but not judged – is very powerful.

Friends and family: provided there is sufficient and genuine trust, then this can be a powerful support network.

Work colleagues: much as above, with trusted colleagues.

Social groups: one of the more interesting social networks that has grown up over recent years is Meetup. It's mostly used by single people, but not exclusively so. Its purpose is social outings and meetings. It is international, and most towns have groups. You can meet up for meals, walks, and general social interaction. There are also many specialist groups too, perhaps focusing on photography or attending philosophical discussions. Group organisers welcome newcomers, and you quickly realise that many people are there on their own, seeking company. It's not a dating site, although inevitably relationships do form. And of course, there are many other groups to consider too – perhaps your local choir, badminton group and so on.

Exercise: Participating in yoga or Pilates; signing up for adult education learning via evening classes; or joining courses will also introduce you to other people. And the regularity of a weekly class starts to build a routine.

Pets: If you like animals and can keep them, then get yourself a pet. Animals are great for unconditional love.

Activity

Create a mind map of the different networks you already have and that you can possibly tap into. All you need is a piece of paper and a pencil. I suggest that you write your name at the centre of the page. Then draw lines from there that link to different groups you are already involved in – and write them down, separately, each in its own setting. Or perhaps you draw a line to interests you have. Allow yourself to make this as simple or complex as you wish. There are no right or wrongs.

The purpose of an activity like this is to bring to your awareness what your complete network might look like – and how you might grow it in a way that best works for you.

Chapter 52

Shape, soften and flex your armour to respond the way you want

The child who is punished for crying will find a way to repress his behaviour. Allow yourself to let the tears flow again.

There's a very common phrase that I am confident you will instantly recognise: "Big boys don't cry."

That admonition, repeated, can have huge repercussions. And I have met many "big boys" as men who seem to wear their lives under a suit of armour, with both a rigid and limited emotional repertoire. Yet there's a perfect riposte to the quote above, which is that while boys might not cry, real men do.

Think of the boy's reaction when punished. The fight, flight or freeze response. He's certainly not fighting back, and it appears he cannot run away, so flight is not possible. Which leaves freeze, when he shuts down. And maybe, over time, he may flop when criticised; he may become numb. He may even fawn, attempting to feel safer by seeking to please and appease the adult.

Earlier in this book, we used the example of Marilyn Van Derbur, a former Miss America, who was regularly sexually abused by her father from the age of 5 to 18. In her book, she describes her chronic muscular tension, and having a body so tense that it is primed to lift a car.

One of the frequently observed outcomes of PTSD is hyper-vigilance – and our muscles, like our minds, can be perpetually on alert – as described above. Locked and tense for years and decades, unable to let go and relax. As we have seen, holding such tension absorbs a huge amount of energy.

To feel a sense of exactly how much energy might be taken up, experiment with this simple exercise.

Put one of your muscles into a tense position. Flex your arm, for example, or stretch your leg. Stretch or tense your muscle as far as is comfortable. Now hold it for 30 seconds, then release. Repeat this a few times. Then just notice how the arm or leg muscle feels – how much energy has been used up in holding that position. You might want to shake the muscle loose, for example.

And now imagine a muscle armoured and ready for action – primed for lifting a car – to use the example above. If your muscles are rigidly locked in place, then how much energy are you using every day just to hold that tension together? It really doesn't bear thinking about. But that has become normal. It has been ingrained in your body, consequently you don't really notice it. It's like putting on weight. Imagine you gain a kilo in weight. And a kilo is equivalent to the weight of a bag of sugar. Imagine how your arm would feel if you carried an additional one kilo bag of sugar around all day.

Earlier, I quoted Petruska Clarkson and her description of body armouring – one which keeps the chest collapsed in a position of resignation, the other in an inflated 'barrel-chested' position of threatened aggressiveness. And so many people hold so much tension in their chests, as we have explored. A recurring theme of this book is to unlock the tension, unlock the muscles, unlock the rigidity, ground in by the impact of the embodied traumatic experiences.

We cannot underestimate the body-mind connection.

And this brings to mind the therapeutic relationship. My therapy sessions have been talking relationships and have never involved physical contact. There are significant transference and counter-transference reasons for this. The therapist touching the client might trigger, for example, traumatic experiences of the client being previously inappropriately touched. (It differs, for example, from coaching, where handshakes are much more common.) Babette Rothschild contends that: "Working with the body does not require touch." In her book *The Body Remembers*, she explores body techniques that do not involve touch.

An alternative approach might be to work simultaneously with a therapist and with a body practitioner. Regular massages will help the relaxation process. Beyond that, treatments such as osteopathy (including cranial and visceral osteopathy), physiotherapy, chiropractic, acupuncture and many others besides might be helpful.

It is frequently the case that healing needs to be applied to both body and mind. Just as with the traumatised mind, so the traumatised body requires care too. James Kepner provides a valuable insight here. Imagine that the individual has developed tense muscles – body armour – in response to traumatic or difficult events they have experienced.

Kepner proposes that touch is not used to break down such rigid armour. It is not about breaking this down, because this rigidity resulted from the body's resistance to the traumatic event. Breaking down such resistance, he believes, would result in the breakdown – and consequential loss – of an essential self-function:

> "We use touch, then, to discover disowned resistance and encourage the use of such resistance in contactful action, that is, to bring it back into useful engagement with the environment."

He's making an important point here. Recognise and honour the resistance.

It's not about breaking down the resistance (which breaks down the self-function) but, through contact, encouraging the body (or part of the body within the context of a whole) to make contact with the environment (person or object) in a newly defined, healthy, meaningful, contactful and safe way.

It is allowing the body – or a part of the body – to connect with the environment in a different, healthier way.

The earlier exploration of yoga proposed a similar approach. Bodily work in yoga is primarily internally focused. Connect more richly with your body internally and allow your body to connect more effectively with its environment in both new and rediscovered old ways.

Remember, people who have suffered from traumatic experiences are not problems to be 'fixed'. The journey, as Kepner suggests, is to encourage them to make contact with themselves, with others and with their environment in newly defined, healthier and more meaningful ways.

Case study

Keith's story: exercise to stay alive

I have reached the conclusion that one of the reasons I am alive today is because of the amount of exercise I have consistently undertaken throughout my life. A 20-year period of long-distance running, followed more recently by a mix of badminton, gym work, running and cycling. I seek to achieve 10,000 steps each day. Having experienced and lived with traumatic and difficult events, I have held a lot of tension within my body. Exercising has been – and continues to be – a way of releasing that energy.

However, one of the things I noticed, particularly in my running career, was a tension between sport and injury. Particularly into my 30s, muscle pulls were increasingly apparent. That, coupled with a burgeoning working career, eventually put paid to competitive racing. It's only since then, when I look back on my running, that I realise that my personal unresolved muscular tensions were core to the diminishing returns I got from thousands of miles of intense training. And these weren't just a lack of flexibility. These were deep-rooted, deeply frozen tensions trapped in time. It is only since I undertook more body work that I have been able to ease out these tensions. The job isn't complete yet and continues to be work in progress.

What exercise did achieve, however, was to provide an outlet for the tension held within my body. I used to think that I was one of those compulsive, addicted runners who needed his daily 'fix'. That certainly has some truth in it. Yet at the same time, I now believe my body was communicating with me. My body needed that outlet to release the tension.

Even today, I notice it. Exercising allows me to ground myself. If I don't exercise, I can find myself getting twitchy and ungrounded. Movement is so important.

Activity

Take some time to think about the type of exercise that is right for you.

Fight: You could try self-defence or take up a martial art. You could join a group or go for 1:1 tuition. Or if you prefer, buy a punchbag and set it up at home. If you use a cross-trainer, work hard on your arms as well as your legs. Or squeeze a stress ball 20 times. Learn to fight. Build up your muscles.

Flight: Perhaps instead of running 'away', try some running that gives you a sense of freedom. Feel the ground beneath your feet and get your lungs working. Or go for a walk. Try cycling – and you can nowadays join many cycling groups of all standards. It is a lovely feeling to feel at one with your bike. Or swim and enjoy the sensation of the water supporting you.

Freeze: Go for a massage to loosen those muscles. Pamper yourself. Or go to yoga or pilates. Stretch your body and breathe as you adopt the various positions.

Flop: Take action, take more control. Move away from acceptance by following the previous suggestions.

Fawn: Let go of the please-driver and appease-driver. Explore conflict rather than avoid it. Hit the punchbag, learn the self-defence.

What exercises can you do?

CHAPTER 53

Rachel's story: Noticing and responding to anxiety and stress in both body and mind

Rachel describes her journey through Covid-19 and the lockdown. She shares her experiences of anxiety and distress, how she notices these within her body and how she uses her 'felt sense' to overcome these feelings.

Applying and teaching yoga became a valuable activity during the pandemic.

Noticing and responding to anxiety and stress in both body and mind

Please give me an overview of the impact Covid-19 has had on you – what happened and/or what is happening.

Since COVID-19's impact on the world, I've found myself dealing with increasingly conflicting emotions. Not necessarily dealing with these emotions very regularly, but when they do arise, they are very intense. If I were to name them, it would be anxiety/distress on the one hand and contentment/gratitude on the other.

COVID-19 has been one of the most uncontrollable events I have faced in my life so far. I've been fortunate enough that I haven't ever experienced significant tragedy or misfortune, at least not while I could comprehend it. I also know I'm a very compassionate and empathetic person.

This combination meant that seeing the effect that coronavirus was having on whole populations without the ability to significantly help people was a very new feeling for me. And a very uncomfortable, almost paralysing one.

Watching the news early on in the pandemic would send me into anxious spirals that I had only previously experienced on a personal level, not as a collective distress for society as a whole. I remember watching the announcement about lockdown and being devastated: I recall holding my head in my hands and not being able to form thoughts, just emotions of complete shock and disbelief.

I've done a lot of self-development work in the past few years to work on my anxiety and stress levels and, fortunately, I can recognise it, manage it and bring myself back in balance much more easily. So I stopped watching the news shortly after the first lockdown was announced, and three weeks after lockdown I made the decision to visit my parents – a decision which was stressful in itself. I live alone and I am very independent, but I felt that being completely alone for what was an undetermined amount of time would be detrimental to my mental health. My parents agreed, and as I had already self-isolated for more than 21 days, I took the risk and visited my parents' home.

But actually, my ability to cope with what was going on – whether that was avoiding the media bombardment, sitting with conflicting emotions, connecting with others virtually, etc. – my ability to cope highlighted my anxiety more.

This is a strange paradox, but the only way I can explain it is that the better I coped, the more anxious I felt for countless other people who might not be able to. It wasn't just a case of checking in with friends and family or those who I felt might benefit from a chat, it was much more far-reaching than that: like a collective sense of distress for society that made me feel helpless.

I am a yoga teacher and, early on, to help others feel more grounded, I offered free online yoga classes. I was also furloughed, an experience that I took advantage of and provided online yoga and wellbeing for people.

For me, the pandemic presented an opportunity. I hold some guilt around this which contributes to the anxiety because several people I know are dealing with life-changing financial situations because of coronavirus, and I am fully aware of the tragedy it has brought to others. So despite the anxiety I've experienced, which still comes in waves sometimes, or perhaps in spite of it, I've thrived in lockdown. I've actually enjoyed it: it took the everyday pressure off to be achieving or running around at 100mph. I had wonderful morning routines; I connected and reconnected with people I love; I know myself better than ever.

So when lockdown started easing, the anxiety I was feeling more widely began to internalise. I got the overwhelming sense that I did not want to return to 'normality'. Whether that was a regular 9-5 office-based routine, rushing to my fitness classes, commuting, not having enough time to myself, or having consistently busy weekends. I was grateful for all of this before lockdown, but a part of me didn't want to return to that normality, and still doesn't – almost like I am anticipating grieving for a way of life I've had for a few months because I feel like it won't survive. To clarify, this wasn't anxiety about contracting the virus as lockdown lifted; it was caused by returning to a way of life that I realised I enjoyed less than the new life I had created.

As a highly social butterfly, the first time my friends invited me to have a socially distanced picnic in the park as lockdown eased, I should have jumped at the chance. Instead, I almost didn't go because I felt physically sick with nerves. The more times I've forced myself out, it's gradually got better, and I know I am the sort of person who can cope and get through these feelings. But again, as I've found the ability to cope and move forwards, I've adopted a different anxiety for others around how they are managing. I would also say there's still some internal anxiety around returning to the regular pressures I felt in my life before lockdown, even though the gradual shift has helped.

I'm feeling more balanced now, but work and returning to the office still provided a source of mild distress. As does the knowledge that we are likely not at the end of the pandemic's impact on our lives. So I guess we'll see where things go from here!

These seem to be strong for you. Have you recognised these [emotions] before within yourself, or have these popped up as something new during the pandemic?

Gratitude and contentment are both emotions I have identified with increasingly in the last year or so, but yes, I would say that since the pandemic I have felt them more strongly. I suppose I've actively felt both in order to cope with the lockdown situation by finding contentment in the everyday and finding gratitude in the small things. So I wouldn't say they are new, but it has allowed me to feel them more deeply and ultimately keep myself in a positive mental state.

Anxiety isn't new to me! I have suffered with anxiety in the past, mainly from the pressure I've put on myself to achieve, succeed, be perfect etc. This caused stress when things (inevitably) didn't always go well. There is a difference in the way I feel it now: as I mentioned, the anxiety now is almost on behalf of others, whereas previously it was definitely something I internalised and was personal to me and my situation.

Distress, however, I would say that is new. I can't really identify ever having been really distressed. I associate that almost with physical pain rather than emotional. I think that could be more related to the human tragedies and suffering that is happening across the world from COVID.

You say: "…the better I coped, the more anxious and desperate I felt for countless other people." What do you consider might be going on here?

My initial reaction is that this is guilt. Feeling a sense of guilt, of shame perhaps, around the fact that I am growing in a world that is dealing with so much tragedy. Reflecting on the question above, I think this is where the conflict comes in: gratitude for my safety and also for how I've coped in the situation, whilst almost simultaneously feeling anxious from the guilt of feeling that way. And that conflict works the other way too: anxious for the wider population and society, whilst also cultivating a sense of gratitude and contentment for my own health and situation.

As I write, I'm reconsidering the idea more closely that this anxiety isn't coming directly from me at all. Yes, it is me feeling this way for a group of other people (and not necessarily even people I know), but actually perhaps what is happening is that I'm almost adopting this anxiety from people who aren't coping as well as me. This is a bit difficult to describe, but as I'm thinking about this, maybe my anxiety isn't genuinely *my* anxiety – maybe it's something that I'm absorbing from others as a wider feeling across society. So not just worrying for others or about how they are coping, but emotionally taking on the collective anxiety that I can feel around me. It's an interesting idea, or it could be a combination of all of the above!

There seem to be two different aspects of anxiety here: from within yourself and from others:

1. **Your personal drivers: Anxiety isn't new to me! I have suffered with anxiety in the past, mainly from the pressure I've put on myself to achieve, succeed, be perfect etc.**
2. **Creeping anxiety from others: this anxiety isn't coming directly from me at all. Yes, it is me feeling this way for a group of other people (and not necessarily even people I know), but actually perhaps what is happening is that I'm almost adopting this anxiety from people who aren't coping as well as me.**

If you allow yourself to relax and allow yourself to experience these two anxieties for a few moments, where do you notice them in your body? Both your personal anxiety and the anxiety from others? Are they located in the same place, or differently? What do you notice?

Interestingly, they are felt in different places. Being present with each of them by imagining myself in a scenario where each anxiety might surface definitely emphasises that whilst I would name it the same thing ('anxiety'), it's clearly not the same thing.

I felt the personal anxiety in my middle and upper chest area and noticed I wanted to take a deeper breath to almost 'unstick' it. The anxiety from others comes up more from my tummy, my gut area and feels like a deep worry – almost anguish I would say. This reminds me of the word distress I described when thinking of what others are going through at the moment – anguish and distress are both suggestive of more physical or emotional pain, as opposed to the personal anxiety, which I would describe more as discomfort rather than emotional pain. I feel there's a difference with that.

As a yoga teacher, what advice and/or body work might you consider for one of your clients who describes these symptoms to you? The anxiety in your chest and the anguish in your tummy? And if your advice/body work involves some yoga, what do you notice (or what have you noticed) if you apply this advice/ body work to yourself? What happens when you allow yourself to notice these within the contact of a 'whole' body yoga session?

I think I was only able to identify these emotions because of my yoga practice and how it has taught me to connect to feeling rather than thinking. If I was giving advice to one of my students, I would encourage them to take a couple of deep breaths, connecting to how the breath moves in and out of the body. Then start to feel where they are in contact with the chair, floor – wherever they are literally grounded. Once comfortable with that, then mentally step themselves into the situation where they feel these symptoms and notice where in the body it is felt... connecting to feeling, rather than moving into thinking or interpreting these feelings. That's how I was able to identify these myself.

When I've been consumed by these symptoms, losing myself in yoga (whether that is the movement or the meditation) is the best way to help myself to process and move through the sensations.

And what are your thoughts on the fact that anxiety is felt in the chest and anguish in the stomach?

I suppose anatomically, the chest is essentially the heart area; the stomach is the gut, increasingly known as the second brain or the source of our instincts. It feels important that the more personal anxiety is in my chest, my heart. Equally, it makes complete sense that the 'adopted' anxiety from others is in my tummy/gut area – like my instincts are picking up on what's around me.

Can you tell me more about "Connecting to feeling, rather than thinking or interpreting"?

For me, this is a key concept in the way I teach my yoga classes because it has been so helpful for me in my own self-awareness. I can physically see the difference in my students when they connect to themselves in this way. Being able to tune into how I'm feeling emotionally and physically brings me to the present moment. It helps move away from worrying about the past or future and brings me more in sync with how I really *am* and helps me to accept it. The key to this is not allowing that feeling to turn into thinking. So, for example, noticing feelings of anxiety and tension across your shoulders might try to turn into a thought process of 'why is that, I'm always so stressed, I hope this yoga class helps, what do I have to feel anxious about, maybe I'm not the only one' etc. When feeling shifts back to thinking or interpreting, judgement (often self-judgement) comes with that. So that's why I try to focus as much as possible on sensations, emotions, feelings: it brings us to the present moment, and encourages us to accept what is showing up for us in that moment, which ultimately increases our self-awareness as we become more in tune with ourselves.

When you have allowed yourself to process through yoga, and to connect with your feelings, how is it for you stepping out of the yoga room and into your everyday world?

One word sums this up for me: clarity. Yoga grounds me. It helps me to get in touch with how I'm really feeling, accept it, and then be able to cope with it. That means that often when I step off my mat and out into the everyday world, especially after a really powerful session, I can feel so light because I'm able to see things from a different, fresh and *clearer* perspective. It's what people tend to associate with the post-yoga 'zen' feeling. But for me, it's not just the 'zen' relaxation aspect, I usually ride this feeling and use it to help me take action, whether big or small.

From your experiences, what advice would you give to others feeling anxieties in their lives?

It's completely normal and can happen to anyone. If there is one thing I could change in the world, it's this idea that we all have to be perfect and strong all of the time. We're human, and we have ups and downs. Being able to accept your own anxiety and then talk to someone you love and trust about it is not weakness; it's strength.

If you can talk, always do. But if you don't feel comfortable talking to someone, then yoga has taught me there is always one thing by your side: your breath. Use your breath like a tool. There's a lot more research coming out now about its powerful effects, so I encourage anyone to start with some simple breathing exercises. Breathing will physically ease anxiety and help with your mind. It's not about doing it perfectly; it's about pausing, grounding and feeling.

PART 9

Live your best life

The last two sections have focused upon how you can be – and what you can do. Combined, these lead to new possibilities of who you can become. Here we are narrowing the focus in terms of specific activities that you might like to do.

In the next chapter, you can find an A-Z guide of passions and activities. You will see that we have suggested eight benefits that you will gain from these – energy, engagement, expression, integration, meditative, movement, soothing and strength. Two or more of these, grouped together, have the potential to significantly help you on your journey from surviving to thriving.

CHAPTER 54

A-Z of passions and activities you can do

Move the body to move the mind.

Having considered acceptance of a traumatic event and developed awareness of the impact it had, it helps to consider specific actions that you can undertake – and here is a list of possible actions you might choose to undertake in an A-to-Z format. There are many more besides, so please do not limit yourself to the suggestions below. These can all be therapeutic in their own way. I make no excuses for the puns in the list below. After all, I have learnt that keeping a sense of humour is very helpful in the recovery journey. It helps to bring reflections up to higher levels of manageability.

While reading through the list below, I suggest you consider the following criteria to speed you on your action recovery journey.

- **Energy**. Does the activity allow you to release energy (including anger) in a constructive, focused manner?
- **Engaging**. Does it engage both mind and hands – and perhaps even your body?
- **Expression**. Does it allow you to express yourself?
- **Integration** (self). Does it promote integration within yourself?
- **Integration** (others). Does it allow you to increase connections with others?
- **Meditative**. Is it an activity that has meditative processes?
- **Movement**. Does it get you moving?
- **Soothing**. Does it allow you to be soothed and relaxed?
- **Strength**. Might it help you to feel stronger as a consequence?

It might be that you undertake more than one of these – and perhaps even create a cycle that you can undertake on a weekly, fortnightly or monthly basis. Do what works best for you. In the next chapter, you will find an Action Plan.

Physical activities

Activity	Benefits
Archery	An activity that engages mind and body, head and hands. And lots of focused attention.
Badminton	Lots of clubs that accommodate all levels. Good for some safe smashes.
Baking/cooking	What a great way to practice integration and bringing things together.
Choir	Join a choir and enjoy singing with others. A super way to get in tune with yourself and be in tune with others.
Climbing	Whether a climbing wall or the great outdoors, you can reach new heights. It is literally gripping stuff – which requires lots of concentration for both body and mind.
Cycling	Feel at one with your bike and enjoy the freedom of the open road.
Dancing	Wonderful way to develop movement and enable expression.
Experimenting	Try something new – which may or not be from this list.
Fencing	On the one hand, you can try fencing, which is a way of looking at defence and attack. Or, for a different kind of fencing, you can paint your garden fence – a therapeutic, mindful outdoors activity.

Gardening	A wonderful, down-to-earth grounding activity.
Golf	Join a club. Or go to a golf driving range and hit the balls as hard as you can. Play a round of nine holes. Many golf clubs have these and driving ranges that don't require expensive membership fees.
Gym	Join the gym. Or get yourself a personal trainer and give yourself a full body workout.
Horse riding	Horse riding is one of those activities that people did when they were younger, but to which they have never returned. Why not get back in the saddle?
Ice skating	Something that many people did when they were younger – perhaps make a return to the ice rink and enhance balance and movement.
Investing	Investing can be risky – so why not start with an imaginary portfolio and see how it fares?
Jewellery-making	Another activity that involves mind, body and focus.
Karate	Never too late to start. Great for self-defence too.
Kick boxing	Clubs can be found all over the place. Step forward to learn the art of defence and attack.
Learn a foreign language	Great for connecting with others – we have discussed online forums. Being able to speak with others in their language is a great way to learn and connect.

Massage	Book yourself a massage. Or perhaps undertake a massage training programme.
Meditating	Practice meditation – make it a regular part of your day. And engage in mindfulness.
Navigation	Learn to read a map and compass – it has been said that the person who never got lost never got anywhere. A great skill to learn.
Origami	Turn a plain sheet of paper into a wonderful, expressive shape. Think of it as a metaphor – if you can turn a sheet of paper into an exquisite shape, what might you become?
Painting	Painting is a wonderful way of allowing unexpressed feelings to emerge. You could try drawing, if you prefer.
Pampering	Allow yourself to be pampered. What works best for you?
Photography	A great way to see the bigger picture. And to keep things in focus.
Pilates	Yoga isn't everyone's cup of tea, so try Pilates instead.
Punchbag	A great home-based activity for channelling and focusing energy.
Quality activities	Commit yourself to undertake activities that will bring a higher quality of living. This is not simply going to the pub or watching a box set. What will enrich your life?
Running	Grab a pair of decent trainers and enjoy the world going by as your fitness levels grow.
Self-defence	Learn to defend yourself – and develop your sense of self-assurance and safety.

Shooting	You could try clay pigeon shooting – another activity that is absorbing for both body and mind.
Squash	Good for alleviating stress. A hard workout.
Swimming	Allow yourself to enjoy the luxury of being surrounded by – and held by – water. A great non-impact sport.
Theatre	People who have had traumatic experiences will have had plenty of drama in their lives – why not join a theatre group to explore drama 'out there' rather than inside? There are many roles needed both on the stage and behind the scenes.
Therapy & treatments	While perhaps not strictly a 'passion', book yourself in for some therapy. Treatments might also include bodily therapy – such as acupuncture or cranial osteopathy.
Toastmasters	Join Toastmasters and learn the art of public speaking. A great way to speak clearly and to be heard!
Upcycling	Rather than just throwing old things out, what can be upcycled to be something new? And that resonates with the post-traumatic journey.
Video-making	We live in the video generation, and more and more people are generating videos that can be cherished for years to come.
Volunteering	Enjoy the pleasure of volunteering for work that helps make the world a better place rather than for money.

Walking	In the city, countryside, along the beach. Or up hills and down hills. Walk on your own, with a friend or join a group.
Writing	Allow your inner thoughts to emerge through writing – try poetry or a course on creative writing.
Xylophone	Learn to play the xylophone – or any musical instrument of your choosing. Join some others too!
Yoga	Really get in touch with your body. Breathe in those new positions.
Zoo	Go to the zoo – you can learn from observing the animals. Combine some animal-watching with people-watching.

CHAPTER 55

Over to you

What you can do

     How you can be

         Who you can become

Each step further away from the past is a step further into the future.

Earlier in this book, we considered the view that the brain's function is to create movement. If you have experienced traumatic or difficult challenges in your life, then movement is crucial on your healing and recovering journey. The purpose here is to consider what more movement you will create.

In the last chapter, we explored different activities that you might like to try. Now you can create robust plans for moving forwards for you to thrive in your life.

Think of it like this. Everything you do to nurture and heal yourself has the potential to move you further away from the memories of trauma. Every meditation, yoga session, bike ride, massage, walk in the countryside, hour in the garden, relaxing drink in a café… each one can take you a further step away from the grip of trauma. Consciously acknowledge that each activity has the potential to create more space from the past.

Each step further away from the past really does take you a step further into the future. You can consciously create your future by attending to your 'wants' and 'needs' right now. These steps can be taken right here, right now. They can be online, in your home, in your garden, in your environment.

You can summarise these into two simple statements, each of which has been explored in previous chapters:

- How you can be.
- What you can do.

Now is the perfect time for you to move forward. To do so requires consciously thinking and then following through on these.

How do you like to think about your time? This will be different for different people, but allow me to provide you with three suggestions:

1. Daily
2. Weekly
3. Monthly

Allow yourself some time to think through which of these timescales is most effective – you might even choose a combination. Using the timings suggested, you can populate these with activities that you are already undertaking. You might then add to them with new themes around being and doing. These are designed to help you increase your movement. Get moving!

Regularly consciously mapping these will help to ensure they have a place in your life. Repeat them, and they become patterns and behaviours. You can create your new normal. You always have a choice in life to do something or nothing. Get moving, take action and good luck!

Daily movements: being and doing

Time	Being	Doing
Morning		
Afternoon		
Evening		
Late evening		
Night time		

Weekly movements: being and doing

	Morning	Afternoon	Evening
Sunday			
Monday			
Tuesday			
Wednesday			
Thursday			
Friday			
Saturday			

Monthly movements: being and doing

	Week 1	Week 2	Week 3	Week 4
Sunday				
Monday				
Tuesday				
Wednesday				
Thursday				
Friday				
Saturday				

CHAPTER 56

Last words: 16 golden tips to accelerate your journey from recovery to health, wholeness and towards future possibilities

"There is always another way". Keith's motto for his journey through life.

1. **Keep breathing**

   Remember to breathe. We do it every day, but how effectively do we breathe? Allow yourself to inhale and exhale more effectively – it can be truly transformative.

   So much tension is often held in the chest and throat areas. Tension constricts and interferes with our ability to breathe in and out.

   People who have suffered from traumatic experiences would often have had to 'swallow' something – or things – that have impacted them. Learning to exhale can be a wonderful way of letting go, of breathing out fully, of releasing 'stuff' from themselves.

2. **Stay grounded**

   Grounding yourself sits closely with breathing, above. Feel the earth beneath your feet. To be more specific, it doesn't matter if you're barefoot in the garden or on the carpeted floor of a high-rise building. Plant your feet on the ground. Feel the solidity. Give yourself a solid base.

3. **Get moving**

   The choice is yours. Walk, run, cycle, go up the stairs, or just empty the bins. One of the effects of the lockdown was to reduce the amount of movement that many people undertook. During the first lockdown, there were huge amounts of activities as people chucked out old stuff, tended to their gardens or redecorated their homes.

In subsequent lockdowns, there was greater acceptance of just sitting. Weight was gained, and conditions known as 'covid bum' and 'bended back' emerged from people just sitting around.

Movement is so important.

4. **Seek out healthy relationships**

Traumatic experiences have the nasty effect of isolating sufferers. Abusive relationships are particularly prone to this. Withdrawing from friends and family and submitting to a controlling partner are not uncommon. Depression and anxiety all too easily lead to staying in.

A therapeutic relationship can be so effective; it can become an anchor point in someone's life. Being able to talk safely is crucial. There are an increasing range of specialist therapies available. Research them, seek them out.

As well as therapy, it helps to have healthy relationships. Be aware of energy vampires; others who might take your energy. Look for – and spend time with – supportive friends and family. Avoid those people who play psychological games; those people who might build themselves up by putting you down.

Good friends are empathic listeners. People who will listen to you supportively and without judgement – and who won't forever be giving you advice or telling you what to do.

5. **Do things your way**

Do those things that work for you on your journey to recovery. Everyone on this planet is unique. Forge your own way and be true to your authentic self.

There are plenty of people who are only too willing to give you advice, 'solve' your problems or tell you what to do. Make sure your filters are in place so that you can:

- Chew on and digest information that might help.
- Swallow what they are saying (only if it's going to really help).
- Spit out and reject what they are saying.

The only person who inhabits your skin is you. Your well-meaning friends or family don't walk in your shoes. You do. They don't have your life experiences. Only you do.

6. Let go

Let go of the stuff that really doesn't serve a purpose any more. Let go of inner judgemental voices; let go of old belief systems; let go of absolute 'musts', subversive 'shoulds' and awful 'oughts'. Allow yourself choices, do things your way, not what your parents (or others) prescribed for you.

Your choices, your decisions, your life, your future.

7. Maintain a sense of humour

Doctors and nurses working in Accident & Emergency departments are renowned for dark humour. It's a way of dealing with truly awful, often life-ending situations. It breaks the tension. Humour can be a great way of bringing us up from the depths of dreadful experiences. It counters the tension. And humour that leads to laughter gets us smiling; it relaxes us and uses different muscles.

8. Keep time in proportion

Recovering from trauma can feel like a long time. It's not unusual to spend a year or more in therapy. Part of the recovery journey is to repeatedly go backwards and then come to the present – a journey of sense-making and understanding. Such time is required to process and bring to closure events from the past.

Consider it in proportion with the length of the time that the trauma has been with you. Perhaps a year or more. Perhaps a decade or several decades. Framing it in this context shows that proportionally your recovery is much more rapid than the length of time the trauma has been with you.

There's a saying in Buddhism that when the student is ready, the teacher appears. There is a 'readiness' in the trauma recovery journey – being able to take on and process topics when you are ready to do so. The skilled therapist works effectively in this way.

9. Don't just listen to your body; feel it too
Really get in touch and in tune with your body. Notice it, attend to it, feel it. What is it saying to you? It's you. Don't disown parts of it. Accept it, all of it. It's who you are. Your body contains you. Your greatest empathic friend is your body, if only you will allow yourself to be in rapport with it.

10. Choices
Every day, in every way, you are making choices. There is little in life that we don't have choice over. Think up your choices, act upon them. Change your behaviours and patterns if you wish.

11. Thoughts are only thoughts
Thoughts are only thoughts. They come and they go. Just as they pop into your mind, so open a window somewhere and let them float away. Never assume – it's said that to 'assume' makes an 'ass' out of 'u' and 'me'. Beware assumptions. Notice those anxieties. Keep them in their place, in proportion. Don't let minor concerns become rolling dark clouds in your mind.
Shift your thoughts. If you're a strong self-critic, then turn down the volume of the critical voice in your head – or tune in to a different frequency. Be kind on yourself.

12. Every day, in every way, things will get better. Never give up
The past is over. Whatever has happened, happened. It's all about the present now, leading into the future. Your future. A brighter future.

13 What is your purpose?
Something that might help is to consider your purpose in life. What is your purpose in life? You might have had a terrible

experience, but how might you be able to use that in a constructive way. Many who have suffered from traumatic experiences go on to helping others in some way.

For me, my life's purpose is to work with others in an empowering manner, to create an environment for people to change their lives for the better. They do it, not me. I seek to create an environment for this to happen. You are responsible for you. I am responsible for me.

14 You don't have a problem that needs fixing. You don't need to be fixed

This might sound slightly contrary, especially if you feel trauma's grip still upon you. As I wrote before, good friends are those who will listen to you with empathy.

You are most definitely not a problem to be fixed. Consider yourself as a fluid process – after all, you are approximately 60% water. Think how flexible and fluid water is – it moves into the tiniest of spaces, and it naturally forms into the shape of whatever contains it.

I long ago realised I am not a problem to be fixed. I like to see myself as a work in progress – ever-changing and definitely not something to be fixed.

Get those creative juices flowing!

15 Choose your way

Your mind is a miracle. Your body is a miracle. You are a miracle. Whatever has happened to you in your past, you are here today. That in itself may be a miracle.

Step forward into a miraculous world of possibilities.

16 The key is in your pocket

We will finish where we started. The key is in your pocket. Go and grab a key. Hold it, grasp it and open the doors to your future.

The answers lie within.

You are the key.

My commitment to continue moving beyond trauma

My commitment to me to grow beyond trauma that happened in the past	
What I am doing to continually move forwards	
How I am being to continually move forwards	
My key affirmation	
Signed	
Date	

References

Chapter 1
Matsakis, A., 1996. *I can't get over it: a handbook for trauma survivors*. 2nd ed. Oakland, CA: New Harbinger Publications. [P.2]

PTDSUK, 2020. *Post Traumatic Stress Disorder Explained* [online] Available at: https://www.ptsduk.org/what-is-ptsd/ptsd-explained/ [Accessed 5 January 2022]

Chapter 2
Bridgland, V., Moeck, E., Green D., Swain, T., Nayda, D., Matson, L., Hutchison, N., Takarangi, M., 2021. Why the COVID-19 Pandemic is a Traumatic Stressor. *PLOS ONE*. Available at: https://journals.plos.org/plosone/article?id=10.1371/journal.pone.0240146 [Accessed 5 January 2022]

PTSD UK, 2020. *Post Traumatic Stress Disorder Explained* [online] Available at: https://www.ptsduk.org/what-is-ptsd/ptsd-explained/ [Accessed 5 January 2022]

Chapter 4
BBC News, 2020. *Coronavirus: Domestic violence 'increases globally during lockdown'*. [online] Available at: https://www.bbc.co.uk/news/av/world-53014211 [Accessed 5 January 2022]

Office for National Statistics. 2020. *Domestic abuse prevalence and trends, England and Wales: year ending March 2020* [online] Available at: Domestic abuse in England and Wales overview – Office for National Statistics (ons. gov.uk) [Accessed 13 July 2021]

Sutherland, J., 2020. *Crossing the line: lessons from a life on duty*. London: Weidenfeld & Nicolson. [Pp. 75-76]

World Health Organization. 2020. *Female genital mutilation*. [online] Available at: https://www.who.int/news-room/fact-sheets/detail/female-genital-mutilation [Accessed 5 January 2022]

Van Derbur, M., 2012. *Miss America by day: lessons learned from ultimate betrayals and unconditional love*. Denver, Co: Oak Hill Ridge Press. [P.26]

Chapter 5
Enders, G., 2017. *Gut: the inside story of our body's most under-rated organ*. Scribe: London. [Pp. 10-12]

Levine, P., 2008. *Healing trauma: a pioneering program for restoring the wisdom of your body.* Boulder, Co: Sounds True. [Pp. 71-72]

NHS, 2020. *Constipation.* [online] Available at: https://www.nhs.uk/conditions/constipation/ [Accessed 5 January 2022]

Chapter 6

Graber, K., 1991. *Ghosts in the bedroom: a guide for partners of incest survivors.* Deerfield Beach, Flo: Health Communications. [P. 3]

Chapter 7

Herman, J., 2001. *Trauma and recovery: from domestic abuse to political terror.* London: Pandora. [Pp. 156]

Chapter 9

Enders, G., 2017. *Gut: the inside story of our body's most under-rated organ.* London: Scribe. [Pp.131-2]

Kline, N., 1999. *Time to think: listening to ignite the human mind.* London: Cassell Illustrated. [P. 74]

Van der Kolk, B., 2014. *The body keeps the score: mind, brain and body in the transformation of trauma.* London: Penguin. [P. 45]

Chapter 10

Milmo, C., 2010. C. Milne. Deaf diplomat loses fight with Foreign Office over posting. *Independent,* [online] 1 November.

Available at: https://www.independent.co.uk/news/uk/politics/deaf-diplomat-loses-fight-with-foreign-office-over-posting-2121832.html [Accessed 5 January, 2022]

Chapter 12

Fisher, J., 2017. *Healing the fragmented selves of trauma survivors: overcoming internal self-alienation.* Abingdon: Routledge. [P. 63]

Chapter 13

Clarkson, P., 2004. *Gestalt counselling in action.* 3rd ed. London: Sage. [Pp. 51-52]

Joyce, P. and Sills, C., 2010. *Skills in gestalt counselling & psychotherapy.* London: Sage. [Pp. 119-120]

Chapter 15

Bourne, E., 2015. *The anxiety and phobia workbook.* 6th ed. Oakland, CA: New Harbinger Publications [Pp. 277]

Chapter 17
Levine, P., 1997. *Waking the tiger: healing trauma.* Berkeley, Ca. North Atlantic Books. [P. 41]

Chapter 18
American Psychological Association, 2020. *APA dictionary of psychology.* [online] Available at: https://dictionary.apa.org/dissociation [Accessed 5 January 2022]

Fisher, J., 2017. *Healing the fragmented selves of trauma survivors: overcoming internal self-alienation.* Abingdon: Routledge. [Pp.4-5]

NHS, 2019. *Dissociative disorders.* [online] Available at: https://www.nhs.uk/mental-health/conditions/dissociative-disorders/ [Accessed 5 January 2022]

Chapter 19
Gallwey, T., 2000. *The inner game of work: overcoming mental obstacles for maximum performance.* London: Orion Business Books. [Pp. 4-18]

Chapter 20
Lawton, S., 2019. *Skin 1: the structure and functions of the skin. Nursing Times* [online]. [Accessed 5 January 2022]

Van der Kolk, B., 2014. *The body keeps the score: mind, brain and body in the transformation of trauma.* London: Penguin. [P. 96]

Chapter 21
Goleman, D., 1995. *Emotional intelligence: why it can matter more than IQ.* London: Bloomsbury.

Chapter 23
Mind, 2020. *Dissociation and dissociative disorders* [online]. Available at: https://www.mind.org.uk/information-support/types-of-mental-health-problems/dissociation-and-dissociative-disorders/causes/ [Accessed 5 January 2022]

Levine, P., 1997. *Waking the tiger: healing trauma.* Berkeley, Ca: North Atlantic Books. [p. 101 & 103-104]

Chapter 24
Koch, L., 2012. *The psoas book: 30th anniversary revised edition.* Felton, Ca: Guinea Pig Publications. [Pp. 42-44]

Northrup, C., 2020 *Why your psoas muscle is the most important muscle in your body* [online]. Available at: https://www.drnorthrup.com/psoas-muscle-vital-muscle-body/ [Accessed 5 January, 2022]

Chapter 25
Kepner, J., 1987. *Body process: a gestalt approach to working with the body in psychotherapy*. Santa Cruz, Ca: Gestalt Press. [Pp. 169-170]

Chapter 28
Gray, J., 1992. *Men are from Mars, women are from Venus*. London: Thorsons. [P.25]

Rogers, C., 1961. *On becoming a person: a therapist's view of psychotherapy*. 2004 Ed. London: Constable [P. 330]

Part 5 Introduction
Herman, J., 2001. *Trauma and recovery: from domestic abuse to political terror*. London: Pandora. [Pp. 133-213]

Chapter 30
Kübler-Ross, E. & Kessler, D., 2005. *On grief and grieving: finding the meaning of grief through the five stages of loss*. London: Simon & Schuster.

Chapter 32
Beisser, A., 1970. *The paradoxical theory of change*. [online] Available at: https://www.gestalt.org/arnie.htm [Accessed 5 January 2022]

Chapter 35
Army, 2015. *The army leadership code: an introductory guide*. [online] Available at: https://www.army.mod.uk/media/2698/ac72021_the_army_leadership_code_an_introductory_guide.pdf [Accessed 5 January 2022]

Chapter 36
Stout-Rostron, S., 2014. *Business coaching international: transforming individuals and organisations*. 2nd ed. London: Karnac. [Pp.238-241]

Chapter 39
Gendlin, E., 2007. *Focusing*. New York: Bantam Books. [Pp. 37, 86]

Strozzi-Heckler, R., 2014. *The art of somatic coaching: embodying skillful action, wisdom and compassion*. Berkeley, Ca: North Atlantic Books. [P. 112]

Chapter 40
Soosalu, G, & Oka, M. 2014. *Neuroscience and the three brains of leadership*, mBRAINING. [online] Available at: https://www.mbraining.com/mbraining [Accessed 5 January 2022]

Chapter 41
Nestor, J., 2020. *Breath: the new science of a lost art*. London: Penguin Life. [P. xx]

Chapter 43
Parsloe, E. and Wray, M., 2007. *Coaching and mentoring: practical methods to improve learning*. London: Kogan Page. [P. 22]

Chapter 44
Metcalf, L., 2006. *The miracle question: answer it and change your life.* 2nd ed. Bancyfelin: Athenaeum Press. [P. 5]

Chapter 46
Stuart-Smith, S., 2020. *The well gardened mind: rediscovering nature in the modern world. London:* William Collins. [P. 65]

Chapter 50
Zimmer, C., 2013. How many cells are in your body? *National Geographic,* [online] 23 October. Available at: https://www.nationalgeographic.com/science/article/how-many-cells-are-in-your-body [Accessed 5 January 2022]

Chapter 52
Kepner, J., 1999. *Body process: a gestalt approach to working with the body in psychotherapy*. Santa Cruz, CA: Gestalt Press. [Pp. 76-77]
Rothschild, B., 2000. *The body remembers: the psychophysiology of trauma and trauma treatment*. Los Angeles, Ca: Norton. [P.xiv]
Van Derbur, M. 2012. *Miss America by day: lessons learned from ultimate betrayals and unconditional love*. Denver, Co: Oak Hill Ridge Press. [P. 521]

Index

About Keith Nelson

Keith Nelson has coached others for over 25 years, and believes that we never stop learning and growing. He also trains others to become coaches and provides supervision for coaches around the world. Keith is Programme Director at the Møller Institute at Churchill College, University of Cambridge

Listening to thousands of hours of clients' stories have led to him writing this book. He has become increasingly aware of the volume of traumatic experiences that people have experienced in their lives. Too often this remains unresolved and leaves them functioning well in some areas, but severely hindered in others. At the same time, he has spent many years living with – and working through – his own traumatic memories. During the first lockdown in the pandemic last year, he concluded that trauma is far too isolating – and by sharing his experiences, together with other case studies – was the best way to increase connectivity and fulfil his life's purpose to help change the world for the better.

His mantra for life is that 'there is always another way'.

You can email him at keithnelsoncoaching@gmail.com

.

CPSIA information can be obtained
at www.ICGtesting.com
Printed in the USA
BVHW061126110722
641837BV00020B/563